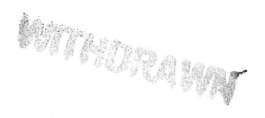

Revolting Bodies?

Revolting Bodies?

· ·

THE STRUGGLE TO REDEFINE

FAT IDENTITY

Kathleen LeBesco

**University of
Massachusetts Press**
Amherst and Boston

LC 2003013815
ISBN 1-55849-428-6 (library cloth edition); 429-4 (paper)

Designed by Jack Harrison
Set in Sabon with Gill Sans display by Binghamton Valley Composition
Printed and bound by The Maple-Vail Book Manufacturing Group

Library of Congress Cataloging-in-Publication Data
LeBesco, Kathleen, 1970–
Revolting bodies? : the struggle to redefine fat identity / Kathleen LeBesco.
p. cm.
Includes bibliographical references and index.
ISBN 1-55849-428-6 (lib. cloth ed. : alk. paper) — ISBN 1-55849-429-4 (paper : alk. paper)
1. Obesity—Social aspects. I. Title.
RC628 .L36 2004
362.1'96398—dc21
2003013815

British Library Cataloguing in Publication data are available.

Contents

Acknowledgments

This book was fueled by excitement and pain, frustration with the way things are and imagination about the way things could be, and the none-too-occasional Ben and Jerry's sugar rush. Much personal and professional support has been provided to me during this period of research and writing, and many thanks are in order for the insights of my colleagues, friends, and family.

For early-inning encouragement and guidance, I thank Leda Cooks, Lisa Henderson, Jane Blankenship, and Barbara Cruikshank; their critical eyes and thoughtful feedback were invaluable in helping me to develop the project. Friends and former colleagues in the Department of Communication at the University of Massachusetts Amherst and elsewhere engaged me in lively intellectual discussions and have helped to keep my flesh happy as well. I am especially indebted to Tami Battin, Margaret Burggren, Melissa Click, Justine Dymond, Louis Faassen, Julie Frechette, Paula Gardner, Meg Honsinger, Nina Huntemann, Nancy Inouye, Kembrew McLeod, Laurie Ouellette, Saila Poutiainen, Katherine Sender, Tim Shary, Alissa Sklar, and Karen Wolf-Wilkins. Also, W. E. B. Du Bois librarians Emily Silverman, J. Mike Davis, and Jill Ausel were of great assistance to me in locating references for the project.

Parts of several chapters originally appeared elsewhere. Portions of the introduction and chapter 7 first materialized within the editor's introduction and the chapter "Queering Fat Bodies/Politics" in *Bodies Out of Bounds: Fatness and Transgression*, edited by Jana Evans Braziel and Kathleen LeBesco. Copyright © 2001 by The Regents of the University of California. Reprinted by permission of the University of California Press. Chapter 8 was published in slightly different form as "Revolting Bodies: The Resignification of Fat in Cyberspace" in *Technospaces: Inside the New Media*, edited by Sally R. Munt (London; New York: Continuum, 2001). Reprinted by permission of The Continuum International Publishing Group.

A 2001 Junior Faculty Leave generously granted by Marymount Manhattan College afforded me the time to work on the manuscript. I am grateful to department chair David Linton as well as deans Ashim Basu, Ann Jablon, and Dawn Weber for their support. Colleagues including Sue Behrens, Terri Dewhirst, Leslie Levin, Peter Naccarato, Martha Sledge, Laura Tropp, and Kent Worcester have also provided enthusiasm and encouragement. Librarians Henry Blanke and Tammy Wofsey aided me in procuring hard-to-get Interlibrary Loan materials. I also appreciate the sleuthing of Julie Tokash, my undergraduate research assistant, and the sense of excitement that this work has generated among my students.

I was able to push the project further while a scholar-in-residence at New York University in 2001, sponsored by the Faculty Resource Network. The administrative staff of the network, including Debra Szybinski, Naomi Diamant, and Ella Turrenne, and my fellow scholars-in-residence provided stimulating conversation and helped me gain access to resources. José Muñoz, my NYU faculty research consultant, was also an inspiration. Librarians at NYU's Bobst Library, the Mary Calderone Library of the Sexuality Information Education Council of the United States, and the New School University's Raymond Fogelman Library were also of great help.

Jana Evans Braziel has been my single most reliable sounding board for ideas on fat politics. A number of other scholars and activists concerned with resignifying the fat body have stimulated my imagination as well. I am grateful for the influence of Shelley Bovey, Marcia Chamberlain, Charlotte Cooper, Elizabeth Fisher, Cecelia Hartley, Joyce Huff, Le'a Kent, Laura Kipnis, Petra Kuppers, Antonia Losano, Sharon Mazer, Allyson Mitchell, Michael Moon, Jerry Mosher, Kristin Pape, Brenda Risch, Esther Rothblum, Eve Kosofsky Sedgwick, Sarah Shieff, Sondra Solovay, Susan Stinson, Angela Stukator, Sarah Tillery, Neda Ulaby, members of the FaT GiRL Editorial Collective, and the early movers and shakers of the Fat Underground.

At the University of Massachusetts Press, I appreciate senior editor Clark Dougan for recognizing the potential of this project, and managing editor Carol Betsch for capably shepherding it through production. Readings of the manuscript by Michèle Barale and Esther Rothblum strengthened the work, and copyediting by Lisa Williams polished my words.

I wish to thank my family—Peg Leahy, Kurt LeBesco, and Pauline Franz—for reminding me to maintain a sense of humor about the academic enterprise.

Finally, thanks to John Shields, for endurance, love, and a comfortable writing chair.

Revolting Bodies?

Introduction

The Discourse of Revolt

Are fat bodies revolting? Popular culture would have us believe so, as would theorists who celebrate transgression writ large, though quite different rationales underpin these similar contentions. In the United States nowadays, as in most Western countries with developed industrial economies since at least World War II, fat has had a bad rap.[1] The medical establishment proclaims fat to be a scourge of the magnitude of the bubonic plague, a "national health crisis," with obesity "striking" nearly one-third of adult Americans.[2] Aesthetically, fat is the antithesis of the beauty ideal of the day: tight, lean, and toned. Viewed, then, as both unhealthy and unattractive, fat people are widely represented in popular culture and in interpersonal interactions as revolting—they are agents of abhorrence and disgust.[3] But if we think about "revolting" in a different way, we can recognize fat as neither simply an aesthetic state nor a medical condition, but a *political* situation. If we think of revolting in terms of overthrowing authority, rebelling, protesting, and rejecting, then corpulence carries a whole new weight as a subversive cultural practice that calls into question received notions about health, beauty, and nature.

My primary purpose in this book is to alter the discourse of fat identity within a research context by moving inquiries about fat from medical and scientistic discourses to social and cultural ones, and to replace self-help literature with a different way of looking at, and living in, fat bodies. My interest here stems from experience of and imagination about the possibilities of political relationships forged from affinities, from the performance of self and recognition of the Other both as subject and subjected. According to Patricia Mann, "if we assume the conjecture of multiple dimensions of both oppression and agency within concrete institutional settings, we can seek to construct a fluid micro-politics embracing diverse forms of intersectional agency and struggle."[4] In so doing, this project guards against the propensity to long idealistically for the emancipation of innocent fat people from the bonds of subjection, just as it suggests alternatives to the notion of helplessness vis-à-vis overdetermined social relationships.[5]

This project is unique in that it approaches political struggle and social transformation from a vantage point of cultural studies *and* interpersonal communication.[6] Although much work has been done to note the importance of forms of action which take as their ultimate goal the deployment of particular public policies or laws, for example, less attention has been paid to the kind of interpersonal agency implicated in the smaller, everyday conversations people have which can help troubled meanings to change over time. Mann maintains that interpersonal agency has been around for a long time but has been dismissed as an insignificant basis for individuated forms of action because the task of creating and maintaining psychic connections to others has historically often fallen to women in male-dominated families.[7] So my project is aimed not only at enabling fat subjects to function with agency, but also at recognizing the power of "small talk" or interpersonal communication to accomplish such goals. I am interested in understanding how forms of interpersonal agency may both aid and complicate practical strategies in struggles for social transformation.

Borrowing from Mann, my analysis demonstrates the serious political implications of the everyday decisions people, fat or not, make about how to act in a certain situation, "even when these decisions are not accompanied by traditional forms of political consciousness." Second, the analysis offers a setting for acting as "intersectional agents" in the realm of cultural politics, but more importantly, with regard to institutional notions of health, beauty, and fitness; it pushes us to consider which actions help to perpetuate or eradicate intersectional relations of domination in a given situation. Finally, the analysis "provides grounds for creative and unconventional forms of political organizing and struggle."[8]

I am interested in how language is used to carry out the revolution that replaces the spoiled identity (in Goffman's sense) of fatness—so powerful that even fat people abhor their own bodies—with a more inhabitable subject position. Judith Butler claims that "discourse becomes oppressive when it requires that the speaking subject, in order to speak, participate in the very terms of that oppression—that is, take for granted the speaking subject's own impossibility or unintelligibility."[9] It is inarguable that current discourse surrounding body size and shape has worked to incorporate the protests of fat people against their own bodies; when civil rights are being argued for on the basis of the genetically determined helplessness of fat people, the fat body is effectively rendered uninhabitable. This power of language isn't purely abstract, either; it enacts physical and material violence on bodies.

Butler, following the work of Mary Douglas, suggests that more important than the question of how a particular Othered identity is internalized is the question of why the distinction between inner and outer is maintained.[10] Whom does it serve in public discourse? When you think about it, only Others internalize things (like oppression), thus rendering their *surfaces* invisible; that is how "a body figure[s] on its surface the very invisibility of its hidden depth."[11] Because of my interest in transforming fatness from a spoiled, uninhabitable, invisible identity to a stronger subject position, I reject analyzing internalization, as it is a paradigm that further propels abjection.

Because "the body is alternately sustained and threatened through modes of address,"[12] it is important to me to examine language communities marked by active communication, rather than to glean something about the construction of fat identity from, say, flat archival materials. I am interested in how agency works through language,[13] through interaction, as a means for positioning an inhabitable subjectivity for fat people, and thus I am most compelled to look at the ways in which they address themselves when speaking and writing.

Language, according to Monique Wittig, "is a set of acts, repeated over time, that produce reality-effects that are eventually misperceived as 'facts.' "[14] The communities that I have chosen to investigate for this project are attempting to create and regulate a new social reality through the use of the written and spoken word. Butler believes that language is capable of enacting material change "through locutionary acts, which, [when] repeated, become entrenched practices and, ultimately, institutions."[15] What I appreciate about this understanding of language is that it does not posit some truly representable reality on which language, like a tool, is used; instead, it speaks to the artificiality of the truths we think we know. Such a recognition of artificiality holds promise for the generation of new truths through language. Butler's work suggests to me that we just might be able to talk our way out of anything, even seemingly ensconced fat oppression, because speaking builds subjects.

However, strategies for talking one's way into a subject position are a point of contention among fat activists today. As I explore more thoroughly in later chapters, rationales for preempting the position of the speaking subject among fat activists are divergent: some want to be able to make claims on behalf of *all* fat people, to posit one specific notion of "the" fat experience, while others want only to be able to speak for themselves and frequently articulate concerns about the oppressive nature of fat community demands. One of the things I examine in this book is the range of terms that fat people use and appropriate to redeploy and destabilize categories of the body and devalued categories for fat identity. This necessitates an analysis of the ways in which these uses both recall and displace the very hegemonic categories that enable their existence.

My analysis, inasmuch as it aims to undermine what counts as normal, must guard against the slip into relativistic evaluation of various transgressions. However, we need some way of discerning which actions are truly disruptive of so-called normalcy, and which in fact help to maintain the status quo. Butler suggests that this requires looking at performances *in context* and asking, What performance in what context will help to destabilize naturalized identity categories.

In this project, I examine the ways in which my research subjects are reworking the signs of fatness so that fat is intelligible in a way that befits them. Butler's argument that "if the rules governing signification not only restrict, but enable the assertion of alternative domains of cultural intelligibility . . . then it is only *within* the practices of repetitive signifying that a subversion of identity becomes possible" is vital for understanding that signification never equals determination, and thus the reworkings in specific language communities provide very real possibilities.[16] This is not a way *out*, but a way *in* to gaining the upper hand in signification games, which means gaining the ability to change the rules by which they are played. To threaten and disrupt dominant significations does not mean to be doomed to a perpetually overshadowed pocket of resistance; rather these actions are "a critical resource in the struggle to rearticulate the very terms of symbolic legitimacy and intelligibility."[17] Elizabeth Grosz concurs with Butler about the vitality of these disruptions: "Where one body . . . takes on the function of model or ideal, the human body, for all other types of body, its domination may be undermined through a defiant affirmation of a multiplicity, a field of differences, or other kinds of bodies and subjectivities."[18] I am aware, however, that the process of gaining the upper hand, or redefining fat identity as palatable, will in turn produce its own subset of unthinkable, unlivable, and abject bodies. Subjects are constituted by the processes of excluding and making abject, so I reflect on these processes in the shaping of fat identity. While I examine strategies for transforming (widening) the fat body, I also consider the ways in which this transformation constitutes excluded and abjected Others. Butler's writing on the possibilities of reworking abjection into political agency is illuminating here, as are Grosz's warnings about simply replacing the current standards of health and beauty with different models, while allowing the structure to remain intact.

In the domain of gender identity, Butler claims that publicly asserted queerness is a first step in transforming the abjection long associated with homosexuality into legitimacy. However, she says that one does not enter oneself into public discourse simply to get the upper hand in the same old tired dialectic, but in an attempt to "rewrite the history of the term, and to force it into a demanding resignification." Doing this, says Butler, is crucial to making queer lives "legible, valuable, worthy of support, in which passion, injury, grief, aspiration become recognized without fixing the terms of that recognition in yet another conceptual order of lifelessness and rigid exclusion." While I recognize her goal of deviating from the citational chain "toward a more possible future to expand the very meaning of what counts as a valued and valuable body in the world" as an exceptionally good one for fat politics as well as for queer politics, I also realize that we're just not quite there yet; constituting the fat body in public discourse still involves some measure of exclusion and abjection.[19]

Similar to Butler, Grosz urges us to refuse "singular models, models which are based on one type of body as the norm by which all others are judged."[20] She instead favors a field of body types "which, in being recognized in their specificity, cannot take on the coercive role of singular norm or ideals for all the others. Such plural models must be used to define the norms and ideals not only of health and fitness but also of beauty and desire."[21] Appreciation of this goal does not imply a naive perspective on happy, separate-but-equal assessment of bodies, because the bringing into being of the plural models is itself an inevitably violent and disruptive process. Ultimately, the question boils down to whether or not it is a *worthy* process, and I address this issue in later chapters.

Another question I bring to the project concerns the foundation of fat identity. Can it be conceptualized as "the stylized repetition of acts through time, and not a seemingly seamless identity," as Butler defines gender identity?[22] What difference does the physical immanence of fat make, as compared with the usually-only-assumed physical presence of a specific set of genitals in gender identity? Although fat, unlike gender, *is* written on the body for *all* to see, what kinds of dissonant and denaturalized performances are possible in the assertion of fat identity?

Paralleling Butler's writings on gender identity, I maintain that the act of fat identity is also "open to splittings, self-parody, self-criticism, and . . . hyperbolic exhibitions of 'the natural.' "[23] Another research question, then, is, where do we see these happenings in my selected fat-identified language communities and what are their consequences for the larger process of resignification?

Grosz's work on identity and the body compels another line of questioning for the retheorization of fatness, fat bodies, and fat politics. She maintains that identities, such as race, class, and sex, are not merely independent vectors that intersect with one another in the space of the person; rather, they mutually constitute one another. Grosz urges us to attempt to understand the body through a range of disparate discourses, instead of confining our inquiries to scientistic and naturalistic modes of explanation.[24] This book, then, questions how we can move the study of the fat body out of the natural and life sciences and into the realm of social and cultural criticism.[25] Ideally, other scholars, activists, and individuals will take a similar approach to the project of rethinking fat bodies. Furthermore, if, as Grosz contends, "bodies speak, without necessarily talking because they become coded with and as signs . . . [t]hey become intextuated, narrativized; simultaneously, social codes, laws, norms, and ideals become incarnated," then it is worth considering how these social codes, norms, ideals, and signs present themselves narratively on culturally invisible fat bodies.[26]

One research question that interests me is borrowed from Judith Butler: what are the political stakes in according naturalness to identity categories that are actually *effects* of multiple and diffuse discourses?[27] Also, what political possibilities open up by a critique of identity categories? This book inquires into the political construction and regulation of fat identity, rather than trying to place shared identity as a foundation for fat politics. Following Butler's claim that the body is a discursive production, this book aims to explore how people use discourse to subvert the notion of fatness as a spoiled identity. I contend that this type of investigation promises possibilities for understanding how a flexible, diffuse fat politics can locate its subjects more favorably within fields of power.

A related research question concerns the ways in which categories of body size and shape are regulatory constructs. In this book I look at the ways these categories are used within specific language communities to empower and subjugate fat people. Do categories of body size and shape, when detached from causal, pathologizing arguments about why a body is the way it is, provide subjects any greater room to maneuver in terms of identity? How is it that categories of health and beauty are constantly invoked and, in turn, refused by those interested in recontextualizing the fat body? Is it possible to explain how multiple discourses converge at the site of fat identity, in order to make that simple category of fatness forevermore a troubled one?

My investigation details the ways in which rhetorical communication strategies in public discourse create, police, and destroy essential "fat" bodies. Such rhetorical struggle is evidenced in discourse processes including "the symbolic meanings of key terms . . . [and] the strategic options for exerting control over interaction and relationships."[28] This introduction defines key terms, rationale, purpose, and history of the project. In addition, I establish the central questions that guided it. I envision the book as a dialogue between narratives of fat identity and theories of the politics of communication, a dialogue that aims to transform both.

Chapters 1, 2, and 3 provide a review of literature relevant to an exploration of possibilities for fat-positive identity performances and narratives. I ground this study in several areas of literature: work on identity politics, including considerations of identity politics of gender, race, and queerness; affinity politics and the notion of "playful subjectivity"; performativity; research on the social construction of the body, with particular attention to the ways in which historical and cultural position differentially constructs the fat body; studies of subversion of hegemonic ideas in Western medicine about the dangers of fatness; and work on ideas of beauty and sexual attractiveness. A review of this literature explains how the renegotiation of fat identities can be undertaken by people, both subjects and subjected, who challenge and maintain popular understandings of nature, health, and beauty and, in so doing, alter their individual and collective relationships to power.

Chapter 4 examines how, in the United States, the bearer of a fat body is marked as a failed citizen, inasmuch as her powers as a worker, shopper, and racially "desirable" subject are called into question. I also discuss similarities between early eugenics campaigns and contemporary well-funded diet crusades.

In Chapter 5, I focus on debates about the political significance of newly available fashions for fat(ter) women. Perspectives which mark the development of products for a fat market as revolutionary, in that they alter the material conditions of a heretofore underserved population, are compared with views that position the opening of fat markets more as a new opportunity for marketers to produce profit than as a harbinger of sociopolitical change.

Chapter 6 explores a number of key popular culture depictions of fatness as a disabling condition. Analyses of the feature film *What's Eating Gilbert Grape?* and an episode of *The Simpsons* shape my evaluation of the state of fat bodies in contemporary popular culture and begin to suggest that fat activists might do well to shadow disability scholars and activists in terms of borrowing cultural frameworks and political tactics.

In chapter 7, I continue the theme of fat rehabilitators as would-be scavengers, by showcasing similarities between queer rhetoric and fat activist discourse. Both share the burden of public attention to the search for a cause of their deviance, and both share the experience of stigmatization that results from the perception of deviance. The chapter examines how the issue of "outing" is understood in both fat and queer circles, and finally considers how the work of fat and queer resignification may be at odds when faced with sizism in queer communities.

Chapter 8 presents an analysis of the ways in which virtual conversations work to resignify fatness in on-line communities. Using critical ethnography, I assess the narratives offered by fat-identified disembodied bodies to suggest how alternative narrative technologies might be useful in changing what counts as political struggle. I demonstrate to what extent self-motivated users appropriate the power of reinvention over against the systems of meaning which contain them, and I pay particular attention to the ways in which the Internet provides or fails to provide possibilities for the development of politically active communities united by affinity, rather than by shared essential identities.

Chapter 9 concludes the book by considering the political efficacy of claiming innocence relative to the state of being fat. This discussion of the long-term ramifications of eschewing bodily agency—in effect, letting biological determinism run rampant—should become influential in fat political practice.

1

. . . .

Organization and Embodiment:
Politicizing and Historicizing Fatness

I am interested in new strategies for playing games of identity wherein pleasure can be taken by and in fat bodies.[1] Following Patricia Mann, it is worth considering to what extent political struggle over the meaning of fat is "buil[t] upon the facts of cultural intersectionality."[2] We can now easily recognize that an actor is as impossibly "simply fat" as she is "simply white" or "simply woman." This lesson, however, was learned the hard way after notable attempts by certain social and political groups to organize their membership by shared, irreducible, and unchanging essential characteristics. It is useful to examine recent physical identity–based political movements of race and gender (e.g., Black Nationalism and second-wave feminism) in order to understand more about the genesis of fat identity politics. It is also necessary to consider the strategy contributions of queer theory and activism to fat politics, a connection documented by Sedgwick and Moon and marked by the possibilities of organizing around conflicted identities.[3] These histories help to illuminate my analysis of what it means to stake a claim to fat identity under very narrow conditions of acceptable subjectivity. They also begin to explain how political subjectivities are constituted in part by the varying values placed on certain bodies in different cultures at different times. I intend to demonstrate how the lived experience of fatness inhabits the same space as, and yet diverges from, other influential subject-marking experiences, like the embodiment of race and sexuality.

With the 1953 publication of Simone de Beauvoir's groundbreaking book *The Second Sex* came the suggestion of a number of social and political changes deemed necessary for women's liberation. De Beauvoir can be applauded for her recognition of sexism as similar to other forms of oppression, but her attempt to describe the situation of *women in general* unfortunately propelled forward the conflation of "woman" with "a small group of women—namely, white middle-class heterosexual Christian women in Western countries."[4] Indeed, in making the assertion that women have done little to incapacitate the institutions that participate in women's oppression, de Beauvoir declares that women are "unlike other oppressed groups—for example, Blacks, Jews, workers."[5] Such a contention holds the categories of "woman" and "black," for instance, to be mutually exclusive; so what of the black woman? She falls through the cracks of de Beauvoir's scheme, much as women of color, lesbians, and working-class women fell through the cracks of the women's liberation movement of the 1970s.

Elizabeth Spelman contends that any attempt to provide an account of the treatment and experiences of women should be viewed with suspicion if such an account is based on only one group of women.[6] This kind of exclusiveness limits the efficacy of political struggle by erasing the potential contributions of people who don't fit easily within the group's confines. Instead, Spelman strives to explain ways in which the notion of woman can be de-essentialized and, accordingly, ways in which women can lay claim to their own subjectivities (multiple, partial, and contradictory) as they organize politically based on ambiguities rather than shared, essential traits. Spelman claims that

> if the meaning of what we apparently have in common (being women) depends in some ways on the meaning of what we don't have in common (for example, our different racial or class identities), then far from distracting us from issues of gender, attention to race and class in fact helps us to understand gender. In this sense it is only if we pay attention to how we differ that we come to an understanding of what we have in common.[7]

She suggests that by owning up to "the variability in the creation of 'women' across and within cultures," by taking responsibility for women's complicity in domination, our ability to act in concert with others, while using our differences as strengths rather than liabilities, will be strengthened.[8] Though many believe that the women's movement has fallen short in this regard, an understanding of the negotiation of fat subjectivity can be further strengthened by investigating political struggle that has engaged the contested and contradictory identities of its participants—queer activism.

Judith Butler criticizes the underpinnings of identity politics, which "assume that an identity must first be in place in order for political interests to be elaborated and, subsequently, political action to be taken."[9] Butler argues instead that the doing of the deed constructs the deed/political act, not the other way around. Queer activists and theorists propose forms of political action which recognize individuals both as subjects with the capacity to act and as subjected to larger forces over which they have less control. For the project at hand, one of the more appealing things about queer theory is its claim that insistent and articulate "rhetoric can control discourse."[10] What can it mean to speak publicly about practices and persuasions that are normatively inscribed with evil meanings, as many queer activists do? Queer theorists contend that such public performance of "perversion" allows sexual subjects to play a part in the ways in which they are inscribed with meaning; to enter themselves into discourse, if you will. As Sarah Schulman warns, "we're wasting our lives being careful."[11]

One queer activist group in particular that exemplifies the potential for the creative and polyvocal practice of cultural politics is the Lesbian Avengers, whose members play with their "selves" loudly and visibly in an attempt to work the meanings ascribed to them to their liking and to their best advantage. A joyful sense of the creatively outrageous is ever present in the Lesbian Avengers' fire-eating, baton-twirling direct-action political organizing. They strive for innovation, shunning hackneyed, out-of-date strategies. Indeed, the authors of the Avenger handbook seem to have abandoned abstract theoretical discussion and false polarities, instead recognizing that members of their audience (other Avengers and wanna-bes) identify themselves diversely both inter- and intrapersonally.

Their radical rhetoric of sex, following Gayle Rubin, "identif[ies], describe[s], explain[s], and denounce[s] erotic injustice and sexual oppression."[12] Still, the exclusive mention of "Lesbian" in the title of the group may raise a flag for some; does their recruitment of lesbians posit the sexual essentialism so common in identity politics? The Avengers steer clear of this problem by making no claims about the fundamental nature of lesbianism; instead, Lesbian Avengers, say, "Imagine what your life could be. Aren't you ready to make it happen? WE ARE. If you don't want to take it anymore and are ready to strike, call us."[13] They leave it up to the callers, the potential activists, to decide what the "it" is that they're not willing to take anymore. They urge imagination and inventiveness in anti-essentialized political action. They encourage playing with one's self.

The persistence of the "Lesbian" title might be explained, following Eve Kosofsky Sedgwick, "not in the first place because of its meaningfulness to those whom it defines but because of its indispensableness to those who define themselves against it."[14] But why would a political group that seeks to dismantle false polarities willingly select a name that lends itself so easily to a lesbian/non-lesbian dichotomy? Are the Lesbian Avengers actually caught up in the same political arena where dangerously essentializing liberal and nationalist political projects exist?

Perhaps Lisa Duggan would step in here to emphasize a "new elasticity in the meanings of 'lesbian' and 'gay' " whereby "the notion of a fixed sexual identity determined by a firmly gendered desire beg[ins] to slip away." Instead of being an identity group, the queer community of Lesbian Avengers "is no longer defined solely by the gender of its members' sexual partners. This new community is unified only by a shared dissent from the dominant organization of sex and gender." Duggan would recognize the Lesbian Avengers as having staked out a new stance of queer opposition constituted by this dissent, and would see in their stress on constant innovation that their "actual historical forms and positions are open, constantly subject to negotiation and renegotiation."[15]

Queer affinity groups (organized by a desire to work or play together, rather than on the basis of a shared identity) like the Lesbian Avengers show promise in terms of allowing individuals to inscribe themselves with meanings over against dominant inscriptions. By exuberantly saying what they do, affinity groups use rhetoric to enter themselves into discourse in significant ways that demonstrate that even small collective actions can make important differences. In a political climate where the comfort of some is predicated upon the silence of others, queer theory encourages us to play with our selves, and to make a joyful noise in the doing.[16]

My investigation of the politics of fat identity finds its roots in this kind of controversy over essentialized identity politics in queer theory, with important implications for communicative bodies. An essentialist position on fat identity can take a biological or sociocultural perspective; the common theme is the idea that the condition of fatness is necessary, could not be otherwise, or is the outcome of some essential (usually failure-related) cause. Whether tracing along a biological path to bad genes or horrible hormones, or along a social path to traumatic childhood experience, proponents of essentialist positions argue that fat identity is the unfortunately inevitable outcome of a causal relationship with some original variable gone awry. Of course, not all essentialist positions are anti-fat; some prefer to focus on the present fact of fatness and the impossibility of changing it and to use this resignation as a platform for civil rights in acceptance movements.

In contrast, an anti-essentialist position on fat identity does not attempt to reveal causal factors; instead it focuses on the ability of human actors to participate in the creation of meaning (including the meaning of material bodies) through the discursive processes of communication and politics. Many examples of such fat activism and discursive negotiation exist, and others are emerging: individuals involved in NAAFA (National Association to Advance Fat Acceptance) and the former Fat Underground; Roseanne, who hosted a "Large and Luscious Beauty Contest" on her daytime syndicated show; other actors, such as Camryn Manheim, who won an Emmy for her work on *The Practice*; and more important, individuals from varied sociopolitical, economic, and educational backgrounds are all invested in projects of fat resignification.[17] It is my hope that scholars interested in corpulence will begin to work through questions of how essentialism functions in the pursuit of effective political struggle, and how people understand themselves via shifting, fabricated locations, tolerating their changes in identity as they cross borders to know and create themselves in acts of agency and resistance.[18]

I hope to have initiated here a different theorization of fatness and fat politics. By *queering* corpulent bodies/politics, perhaps we can equally resist dominant discursive constructions of fatness, while opening new (and playful) sites for reconstructing fat bodies through a lens that examines the corporeal alongside the material, the racial, and the sexual as mutually constitutive elements.

Underlying this project is an understanding of communication as the primary process by which identities are negotiated and narratives are constructed—a process with the potential to alter power relations in meaningful ways. I take my cue from interrogations of essentialism in queer theory and performance studies, which suggest that identities are never merely descriptive; rather, they are strategically performed. Cindy Patton treats identities as a series of "rhetorical closures"—persuasive conclusions about who one is—that connect and reconnect with political strategies and alliances to stage political claims; she suggests that we reconsider identity to see how it is used in everyday life, where the struggle to control the rules of identity construction is played out.[19] As with communication from a position of queer identity, fat identity, however performative, has every possibility and probability of being read as a descriptive admission to what current Western mainstream standards imagine as grotesque perversion. A consideration of the ways in which fat identities alter the modes for staging politics (rather than merely representing yet another aesthetic choice) highlights the importance of communication as political practice.

Judith Butler claims that performativity must be understood "not as a singular or deliberate 'act,' but, rather, as the reiterative and citational practice by which discourse produces the effects that it names."[20] Thus, I investigate not an isolated incident symbolizing fat identity but ongoing discursive negotiations that regulate and constrain the signification of fat bodies. Because these negotiations are ongoing and are often able to be cited as productive for fat bodies, they enable a stronger redefinition of fatness than one-time interventions do.

The fat body is largely invisible in scholarly communication literature. However, on reviewing much of the most recent interdisciplinary academic literature on women, food, and embodiment, I have noticed two trends: first, most focuses on anorexic or bulimic women; second, most imposes meaning onto people's experiences of food and body without considering people's *own* meanings.[21] I believe that these factors perpetuate existing body-image stigmas, which disenfranchise those whose bodily dimensions and experiences do not match the current mainstream ideals of society; but more important, these trends in the literature ignore the lessons to be learned by careful interpretive study of the narratives of other resistant subjectivities.

Much of the literature on women with eating "problems" presents physiological, psychological, or neurochemical explanations for their "abnormal" consumption habits. The small percentage of these writings which are from the social sciences generally project onto women's eating problems a prestructured explanation of women's reaction to body-image pressures. This approach is problematic in that it neglects the (limited) power of women who have particular eating habits to define and create their own realities. In doing so, it fails to endow them with the ability (or, rather, to recognize their already existing abilities) to *change* their realities. Some of the most recent literature that, I think, breaks through this predetermination of meaning incorporates the explanations women hold for their own behaviors, thereby showing emancipatory potential.[22] The danger, I believe, is that this theoretical tack denies the very real exigency that "empowered" women can eat or starve themselves to ill health and even death.

It is important to consider *who* decides what empowerment means: should the agent decide for herself? Or is it the authority of some external source, like Overeaters Anonymous or the academic researcher, which declares her "empowered"? An approach to the study of fat identity that takes subjects' meanings into account as it considers their subjection seems appropriate for dealing with fat-identified people whose bodies do not conform to society's wishes and who therefore do not fit so easily into tight, prestructured explanations.

Unfortunately, even research that puts women with eating disorders into discourse still excludes the fat-identified subject. Research in the "hard" sciences ignores people's own accounts of their experience, while social science replaces the fat-identified subject with a subject whose desire to be "normal" determines her identity. While I do not expect this book, an interpretive study of public communication about fatness, to dissolve the rampant anti-fat sentiment and behavior of many Americans, I do expect that the information it presents will generate another, more useful, way of working toward changing notions of beauty, health, and acceptable sexuality.

Current perceptions of fat are framed by our historical, cultural, and economic position. In a modern capitalist patriarchy such as the United States, fat is seen as repulsive, funny, ugly, unclean, obscene, and above all, as something to lose. As recently as thirty years ago, this notion began to be actively challenged by radical fat activists who argue that our perception of fat is not natural—that it is instead a function of our historical and cultural positioning in a society that benefits from the marginalization of fat people.[23]

In an attempt to debunk an ethnological perspective on perceptions of fat, thus creating political space for the subjectivity of people whose body size does not adhere to society's confining standards, I examine the conceptions of fat held in two quite distinct premodern ages and survey a wide variety of perspectives on fat outside the United States in modernity. My discussion of fat images in Ice Age Europe (particularly in the Aurignacian and Middle Magdalenian periods) and the Hellenistic period of Greece, and my investigation of perceptions of fat in modern Italy, Northern Cameroon, Nigeria, and the Pacific Islands, serves as one way to write into existence an empirical foundation for political action, for with this re-creation of a fat history, fat people can begin to be mobilized.[24] The richness and variety of meanings attributed to body size in both examples demonstrates the *in*consistency of our modern view of fat and lends support to the political project of fat activists who attempt to illustrate the politically marginalizing social construction of fat. Removing the blinders of late twentieth-century America, one can see that fat is a fluid construct that has been used to serve dominant economic and cultural interests, to the detriment of not just the fat people.

Several products of artistic crafts (small, portable objects) have come down to us from the late Ice Age; the earliest of these are plastic human figures, crafted primarily in the middle Aurignacian period (29,000–26,000 B.C.) and later, and to lesser degree, in the middle Magdalenian period (17,000–14,000 B.C.). According to Johannes Maringer and Hans-Georg Bandi, of the over 130 specimens found in the area of Europe from the foot of the Pyrenees to Lake Baikal (which was free of ice in these periods), the vast majority are small statues of female bodies. In describing the realism that is characteristic of most of the Aurignacian sculptures, Maringer states that "any attempt at individualization and portraiture seems to have been excluded, but the female characteristics are often greatly stressed or exaggerated. With few exceptions, they represent naked figurines."[25]

The most famous of these figurines, according to Maringer, is probably the one that has come to be known as the "Venus of Willendorf." Found in 1908, the sculpture

> represents a mature woman with her hair arranged in the shape of a beehive, huge, bloated, pendulous breasts and enormously broad hips; the extraordinarily thin arms rest on the bosom. She has often been called "Venus," but that is rather absurd. . . . The most obvious thing about the figure is its exaggerated corpulence. But . . . it is not unique in that. Indeed, the woman of Willendorf may be considered the classic model of that physioplastic or Rubens type.[26]

This and other well-known Aurignacian statuettes of fat women are marked by an emphasis "on the central part of the female anatomy, in contrast to which the other parts appear to be consciously neglected and the proportions consciously altered."[27] These figurines served as prototypes for later, though highly stylized, statuettes of the Magdalenian period, which were worn as pendants.

Contrary to Maringer's peremptory assumption that to label a fat figure "Venus" is absurd, I find it necessary to consider the historical and cultural location of these figurines. The art historian Laetitia LaFollette contends that the Venus figurines were worn around the hearth by women in a period when body fat was seen as a luxury that permitted the otherwise endangered possibility of human reproduction. White, in a discussion of nutrition and health of Upper Paleolithic peoples, suggests that human nutrition was at its worst in two periods when more people needed to be fed than there were available resources.[28] These periods of highest population density were the Aurignacian and the Magdalenian, not coincidentally the periods marked by a preponderance of "Venus" sculptures. In an age when survival of the species depended on nutrition and fertility, fat statuettes were seen as good-luck charms—as representations (even if exaggerated) of an aesthetic ideal that served a practical function.

White offers a competing notion of the meaning of these figurines for Ice Age peoples. He recognizes that the term *Venus* carries connotations of deity, to the point where the figurines are identified by casual observers as "fertility goddesses." He reminds us, that however, evidence neither confirms nor denies this interpretation, and he suggests a stumbling block to the perception of the figurines as totems:

> even if the notion of fertility goddess is accepted as reasonable, Ucko and Rosenfeld (1972) raise an important question about the fertility issue. All known hunters and gatherers today are much more concerned with limiting rather than increasing their population. It is hard to imagine circumstances in which hunting and gathering peoples would purposely seek to increase population density.[29]

He goes on to suggest, though, that a current understanding of world population problems reveals that "people do not always strive to match their numbers to available resources."[30] White's struggle to understand the meaning of fat figures in these periods indicates the difficulties of interpreting historically and culturally bound information from the position of "outsider." I think, though, that it is important to recognize that the fairly consistent labeling of fat Ice Age figurines as "Venus" is in itself evidence that different historical and cultural conditions allow for quite variable understandings of the meaning of fat. Consider these understandings in comparison with those of a more recent period, the Hellenistic.

The Hellenistic period of Greece offers several statuary representations of various degrees of fat. Though certainly nowhere near the rotundity of Ice Age figurines, Hellenistic statues of goddesses (particularly Aphrodite, goddess of love) and philosophers (predominantly from the Epicurean school) sport bodies that would be considered overweight by today's maintream American standards.

Though many sculptures of Aphrodite have come down from antiquity, Arielle Kozloff and David Mitten claim that none enjoyed the renown of Praxiteles' Aphrodite of Cnidus. This enticing, forbidding marble sculpture depicts a voluptuous nude; but the attention given the statue is what is most impressive: "It served as an object of admiration and pilgrimage for many centuries."[31] Kozloff and Mitten characterize Aphrodite's body as representative of the Classical feminine ideal, with its ample breasts, well-rounded hips and buttocks, and overall full form, yet say that the sculpture never hints at fatness: "Though not the firm, slender form of an adolescent, the soft torso gives no suggestion of obesity."[32] Other sculptures of goddesses, including variations on Aphrodite and Demeter, goddess of the earth, consistently emphasize this fullness and maturity of the female body.

This emphasis is consistent with what Andrew Stewart refers to as the characteristically Greek approach to sculpture, based on a conception of human beauty expressed in terms of geometrical harmony: "Beauty in physical bodies is manifested largely via mass, volume, and proportion. . . . There is a preference for positive form, for volumes that, even though cut into a marble block or scooped out of a lump of clay, grow from the core of the statue and swell organically towards the spectator."[33]

Just as the goddess statues represent well-proportioned massive volumes that swell organically, so do statues of philosophers. Kozloff and Mitten discuss a bronze statuette of an Epicurean philosopher as the most sensitive, sympathetic portrait of the Greek intellectual preserved from ancient times: "The unsettling effects of his girth are especially obvious from the back, where the out-turned feet . . . are widely spaced to steady his weight. From the front, large, flaccid breasts hang heavily over his expansive paunch, and the loose flesh at the inside of his armpits shows the extent of physical deterioration due to both age and indulgence."[34] This heavy figure reflects not the self-indulgent hedonist that later critics claim Epicurean philosophers to be, according to Kozloff and Mitten, but rather "an unsentimental image of contemplation, evocative of an age when the dedication to self-examination and intellectual discipline were considered essential characteristics of a learned man and the philosopher-teacher was among the most respected and influential members of society."[35] It would seem, given the popularity of the philosopher figure in the Hellenistic period, that his representation as a heavy person reflects favorably upon the cultural connotations of fat of that time; a chunky body is used to signify the presence of something good.

However, this leap in understanding must not be made so quickly, as an examination of the contradictory notions of the "ideal" reveals. When discussing various sculptures of Aphrodite, Kozloff and Mitten suggest that their creators seek to associate her elevated status with what is popularly considered beautiful: "Clearly not interested in demonstrating his ability to convey accurately the mundane details of human anatomy, the artist has concentrated instead on creating an image of lyrical beauty worthy of an immortal."[36] Thus, the depiction of a full, heavy body (socially popular at the time) serves to exalt the individual concerned.

Stewart critiques this notion, stating that the exaltation of individuals as heroes or divinities is "not conveyed through 'idealizing': characterization of a subject as better than the average by idealizing him is . . . a product of a quite different outlook."[37] Philosophers and love goddesses, then, are fat not because Hellenistic peoples equate utopia with full bodies; in fact, Greek artists sought to represent as beautiful that which is common, rather than utopian: "Greek artists sought not to construct utopian images, but inquired after the universal and general, the mean which we all mirror and which to a greater or lesser extent can be seen through us. This [is] the 'beautiful.'" The Greeks tried to create more "democratic" images, rather than the idealized utopian representation, of especially popular figures like philosophers and love goddesses, in an attempt to "show them as typical and therefore 'ideal' representatives of Athenian citizen arête," according to Stewart.[38]

Given this controversy over the meaning of fat (or of "fullness," as Greeks might say) in the Hellenistic period, as well as the similar controversy over the meaning of fat figurines in the Ice Age, it is inevitable that one would question how certain meanings have come to take precedence in the discourse on bodies. Though it is possible that both Hellenistic and Ice Age representations of fat are indicative of those cultures' desire for or appreciation of fat, this meaning is seldom recognized.

Other, more modern examples of cultures in which large body size is considered desirable are drawn from (not surprisingly) areas outside the industrialized urban West (namely, the Mediterranean/North African region and some Polynesian locales). In developed countries like the United States, most residents are armed with the financial means to escape social rules and ecological constraints regarding food consumption. Igor de Garine argues that the positive valuation of fat which exists in areas marked by scarcity or irregularity of food supply—"look how much abundance I have"—is replaced by the view that "I'm so safe I can afford to ignore abundance."[39] Indeed, Garine contends, the psychopathological attitude demonstrated toward fat in North America illustrates cultural and class "distinction," in Pierre Bordieu's sense. The militancy of our cultural preference for thin, ascetic bodies likely stems from northern European Puritan attitudes toward sex and food, wherein the fat, indulgent body is seen as anathema to the "proper" embodiment of spiritual devotion, efficient work, and high socioeconomic status. Fear of fat thus "reaches obsessional levels in northern hemisphere Protestant cultures, though is milder in southern European Catholic countries."[40]

For example, Victor Teti writes about perspectives on food and fatness in Calabria, in Southern Italy, during the early part of the twentieth century. Teti suggests, through a detailed examination of literary representations of Calabrian life during this period, that plumpness symbolized wealth and was equated with beauty; in fact, fat was the aesthetic ideal during times of undernourishment. Fat meant strength, health, and resistance to the back-breaking work necessary for survival in this part of Southern Italy. However, after an economic boom in the 1950s improved Calabrian food standards, evaluations of corpulence became negative. It was "only halfway through the 1960s—when food consumer goods finally had been extended to the vast majority of the population—that fat people, becoming more numerous, began to be considered as ill." Forty years later, now that most all Calabrians can afford to be fat, "fatness is no longer a model as when it signified wealth, power, affluence, beauty."[41] I include the example of Calabria not to induce "famine nostalgia," but to suggest that values aligned with different body sizes largely depend on what is difficult to attain in a given sociocultural and historical context.

Many researchers have written about the value placed on fatness by cultures whose members utilize a "fattening process" to ensure distinct cultural identity or fertility or to demonstrate family wealth.[42] The Massa of Northern Cameroon consider fattened males to be beautiful and desirable, moral, powerful, serene, and strong; they engage in ritual collective fattening sessions, institutions that reinforce Massa cultural values and allow the accumulation of status based on local standards rather than on the invasive external cultural forces of the area.[43] Fatness, for the Massa, functions as a way of resisting the aesthetics and work requirement of the modern world.

P. J. Brink contends that the Annang of Nigeria value "women of substance" for their health and beauty. Women are deliberately fattened up in fattening huts before marriage. For many Annang women who are involved in hard manual labor throughout their entire lives, this fattening period is the only time of rest and relaxation they can expect. Because the period of fattening takes women away from the labor force, the ability to fatten a daughter signifies family wealth. It also suggests personal fertility. (Clearly, the relationship between fat and power is articulated quite differently in this instance than in earlier examples.) Brink reports that today's Annang consider the fattening process to be old-fashioned but that it is often used as a treatment for infertility. This, Brink suggests, reflects on the Annang relationship to the economic situation of Nigeria: the shift from agriculture to a cash economy, the instability of oil revenues, and insufficient revenues from other cash crops force people to turn back to subsistence farming.[44] Thus, large body size is valued as a predictor of fertility, which means more workers to aid in the harvest.

A final example of an area in which large body size does not incur the same stigma as it does in the West is in Pacific societies. Nancy Pollock suggests that favorable regard for fat stems from the period of Polynesian evolutionary heritage which required "protection against the cold on the open ocean during the period of voyaging."[45] In addition, cyclones and droughts in the Pacific caused irregular food supply and fostered feast-or-famine lifestyles among island residents; a generous supply of body fat could mean the difference between life and death. Some cultures, like the Nauru, used fattening huts to keep menstruating girls prepared to conceive and produce healthy babies, despite the vagaries of the food supply.[46]

It is easy to comprehend why corpulence would be positively valued in Ice Age Europe, the Hellenistic period of Greece, and modern Italy, Northern Cameroon, Nigeria, and the Pacific Islands: social, cultural, and economic forces *needed* fat. This, however, seems not to be the case in the West today. Explanations for the currently preferred (and ultimately unjust) construction of fat can be found by exploring Douglas's work on "pollution" and Turner's on "liminality"; the perceptions commonly held today of fat as dirty and of the fat individual as liminal blind us to the possibility that fat could be constructed as beautiful, ideal, or desirable. By deconstructing some of the ways in which we think of fat, we can come to understand the heavy body not ethnologically as a naturally negative/bad entity, but as a historically and culturally conditioned effect— and, as such, as one that deserves a fair opportunity to be considered in a more flattering light.

This deconstruction begins by discussing fat as it intersects with Mary Douglas's notion of pollution. Considering the trope of the "fat slob" in modernity, dirt and fat are images that currently go hand in hand. Their connection, though, is not by chance alone. Douglas claims that dirt is disorder. "In chasing dirt, . . . we are not governed by anxiety to escape disease; but are positively reordering our environment, making it conform to an idea."[47] Following this, if fat is considered dirty, then the way we talk about fat *controls* fat—reins in its excesses. The idea that fat is dirty works to reinforce social pressures.

According to Douglas, dirt avoidance is not merely arbitrary; it is creative and well-reasoned. The same can be said for fat avoidance, which posits bodies as evidence of moral codes. "These danger beliefs . . . are a strong language of mutual exhortation. At this level the laws of nature are dragged in to sanction the moral code. . . . The whole universe is harnessed to men's attempts to force one another into good citizenship. Thus we find that certain moral values are upheld and certain social rules defined by beliefs in dangerous contagion."[48] Fat and dirt are connected for political reasons: the concept of fat as polluting can be used strategically to counter status claims by fat individuals.

Douglas states that "some pollutions are used as analogies for expressing a general view of the social order."[49] Her discussion of sexual dangers is meaningful to a consideration of fat as pollution. Douglas gives examples of sexual dangers; for instance, some discourses articulated around sexual intercourse dictate that fluid exchanges are dangerous for both male and female partners, while others indicate that contact with fluid is dangerous for only one partner.[50] These beliefs cannot be interpreted as reflective of actual relations between the sexes, Douglas says. "They're better interpreted as symbols of the relation between parts of society, as mirroring designs of hierarchy or symmetry which apply in the larger social system."[51] This statement can be used to explain beliefs not only about sexual dangers but also about the dangers of dirt and fat.

Though the larger social system promotes certain symbols to mirror its structure, these societal ideas are capable of being changed. Douglas believes that they are in no way stagnant or rigid and questions the person who *absolutely* equates fat with dirt or pollution. Given that societal conceptions are malleable, my goal becomes the reconstruction of fat so that it is not considered bad or dirty, and so that different interpretations of Ice Age and Hellenistic sculptures gain widespread favor. The objective becomes the construction, through language, of an interpretive climate in which true subjectivity can be afforded to fat individuals.

This reconstruction may be difficult to attain, as Douglas indicates when she says that "it is only by exaggerating the difference between within and without, above and below, male and female, with and against, that a semblance of order is created."[52] By making fat bodies "dirty" and "normal" or slender bodies "pure," we have order. The question, then, is why fat bodies, rather than slender ones, are given a negative and damaging social construction.

The rise of the social connotation of fat with something as negative as dirt may be a result of the ascent of Judeo-Christian religions since the times of the Ice Age and the Hellenistic period. Scriptural writings from Deuteronomy and Leviticus (specifically, the abominations of Leviticus) institute a number of dietary rules for religious believers. Douglas states that many of the rules are arbitrary devices used to discipline believers, rather than imbued with religious symbolism. Following this, gluttons, or people who are undisciplined eaters, are in violation of biblical edict and are considered evil. Given the historical condition of the upsurge of Judeo-Christian religions, it is easy to understand how another bad characteristic, uncleanness, gets connected symbolically with fat in modern interpretation. If cleanliness is indeed next to godliness, then one who is unclean (or heavy) is ungodly.

Douglas also discusses conceptions of marginal peoples, a description apt for both fat and unclean people under Christianity's rubric. Marginal people are placeless, left out of society's patterning. Though they are perhaps morally righteous, their status is indefinable, says Douglas. Fat people are marginalized; they are kept from full participation in societal games of health and beauty, in that they are never allowed to win. Douglas claims that "to behave anti-socially is the proper expression of their marginal condition. . . . To have been in the margins is to have been in contact with danger, to have been at a source of power."[53] In this statement, Douglas recognizes the possible connection with power that marginalized people, such as the fat, have available to them if society chooses to construct them in a positive light rather than a negative one. Remember that there were controversies over the meaning of fat in Ice Age and Hellenistic sculptures: was it revered or merely a symbol of the flawed-but-attainable? Modern times tell us that fat couldn't possibly be revered, so it must have been the latter interpretation that guided the artists. However, Douglas subversively notes that this less favorable interpretation comes only as the result of there having been a possibility that it could have gone the other way—that we could construct fat as desirable—but that political necessities precluded this outcome. The important thing to note, of course, is that fat is socially constructed along lines of power.

The power lines in this case, I argue, are those of the Bible. Douglas suggests that pollution dangers "inhere in the structure of ideas itself and . . . punish a symbolic breaking of that which should be joined or joining that which should be separate. It follows from this that pollution is a type of danger which is not likely to occur except where lines of structure, cosmic or social, are clearly defined."[54] Religious power seems to clearly define those lines of structure; it is in light of the historical and cultural condition of the rise of Judeo-Christianity that polluted individuals (here, specifically, the fat) become marginalized. The conception that they are bad is simply that: a conception. It is not a truth that marginalizes them, but a historically appropriate fear that they will gain access to tightly held power.

In light of my interpretation of how and why fat is conceived of as pollution, it is useful to examine the ways in which the lived experience of fat people resonates with Victor Turner's notion of the liminal individual. As one who transgresses boundaries, the fat individual represents an existence that allows for the continued damaging construction of fat people as dangerous or bad. In order to combat this construction, it is necessary to comprehend how it partially consists of the perception of fat people as marginalized, liminal Others.

Fat represents an interesting twist on notions of boundary transgression. The fat individual extends beyond "normal" physical space while still existing within his or her own body; however, physical space is not the only threshold being crossed. The fat individual also transgresses a range of social boundaries (including biblical dictates, as discussed earlier). What does a portrait of such a physical and social transgressor look like? What consciousness accompanies such transgressions for these individuals? And how can their subjectivities be favorably resignified and recontextualized?

Consider the experience of being fat as a rite of passage. Turner, following Van Gennep's 1909 work, demonstrates that rites of passage are marked by the phases of separation, margin (threshold/limen), and reaggregation.[55] Separation consists of behavior that symbolizes detachment (sometimes even literal segregation) either from an earlier fixed point in the social structure or from a set of cultural conditions, or both. In modern fat experience, one might think of the inability of the fat individual to be considered by others (the "normal" center) as a sexual being as an act of separation.

In the liminal period, the ritual subject ambiguously slips through an interim cultural realm, according to Turner.[56] In modern fat experience, this realm might be inhabited by subjects whose meanings for the sexuality of their bodies are still being struggled over; their sexual subjectivity is ambiguous. Meanings are contested; once again, the question is asked: Is fat something to be revered, or is it flawed and thus easily attainable?

In the reaggregation phase, the subject is once again in a relatively stable state and is positioned vis-à-vis others inhabiting the same structure. He or she is bound to act in accordance with the norms and standards associated with the position. This understanding of the reaggregation phase offers some insight as to why most people view fat as naturally bad: seeing fat individuals stabilized within a negative position, accepting the norms that perpetuate their marginalization and mistreatment, might provoke the thought that such treatment is not only deserved but natural. Fat people who have (however uncomfortably) internalized the very standards that oppress them actually assist in their own betrayal by maintaining the idea that this is the way it's supposed to be.

Fat people exist as threshold people, as persons who "elude or slip through the network of classifications that normally locate states and positions in cultural space," only temporarily.[57] Though the meaning of their experience is constantly up for grabs, it is usually grabbed most quickly by societal powerhouses interested in strengthening their own position in relation to all competitors. The meaning of fat is, then, constantly reaggregated in a negative light, made to appear naturally bad. This coup is possible because during the phase of liminality—when fat people are not recognized as fully functioning persons, sexual persons, truly happy persons—they do not aggregate among themselves. They not only do not belong to a "normal" state or set of cultural conditions, they do not generally band together to mobilize in political action (in contrast to African Americans or women, two other traditionally marginalized groups). They are neither in the "here" of the center nor the "there" of the margin; "they are betwixt and between the positions assigned and arrayed by law, custom, convention, and ceremonial. As such, their ambiguous and indeterminate attributes are expressed by a rich variety of symbols in the many societies that ritualize social and cultural transitions."[58]

For fat people, political organization against the domination of the center and against their future unempowered home in the margin is difficult. Turner says that the behavior of liminal entities "is normally passive or humble; they must obey their instructors implicitly and accept arbitrary punishment without complaint. It is as though they are being reduced or ground down to a uniform condition to be fashioned anew and endowed with additional powers to enable them to cope with their new station in life."[59] How, then, can we alter the political landscape that marginalizes fat individuals?

Liminal phenomena, according to Turner, offer a mixture of lowliness and sacredness, of homogeneity and comradeship. Fat liminality incorporates recognition of the mainstream's belief that "more is less" and allows each individual to locate him- or herself on a continuum of "moreness." However, somewhere in the silence of liminality, Turner might imagine that fat individuals begin to recognize one another (and the "normal" rest of the world) as a relatively undifferentiated *communitas* (a communion of equal individuals).

Turner claims that "for individuals and groups, social life is a type of dialectical process that involves successive experience of high and low, communitas and structure, homogeneity and differentiation, equality and inequality. The passage from lower to higher status is through a limbo of statuslessness."[60] The problem with this line of thought is that the experience of liminality for fat people is anything but statusless; it's a training ground for socially accepted subjugation. It is obvious that modern, mainstream conceptions of fat color our interpretations not only of bodies in the present, but even of ancient works of art like the Ice Age and Hellenistic goddess and philosopher sculptures. Turner's hopeful contention that liminal people recognize one another during liminality has little consequence for their empowerment; instead, they are imbued with the construction that they deserve to be marginalized, and then they actually are marginalized. Any plan that assumes that people will organize and does not provide them some kind of socially conceivable forum in which to do it is destined to fail. Following Turner, fat people continue to participate in a kind of pseudo-subjectivity that reintegrates them into the larger social structure as people longing to be objectified; their subjectivity, I argue, is tragically relegated to a status lower than the agency of objectivity. To paraphrase Eve Sedgwick and Michael Moon from their work on Divine, fat people constitute society's "haunting abject."[61]

As long as no one questions the genesis of the idea that fat is dirty, as long as no one questions why the larger social structure benefits from the marginalization of fat individuals, as long as fat people remain complicitous with this larger structure, fat as bad will continue to seem natural rather than be exposed as the social construction that it is. The meanings of artifacts such as the "Venus" figurines of the Ice Age and the goddess and philosopher statues of the Hellenistic period will not be contested; it will be assumed, through today's culturally constructed historical blinders, that fat is something that is now and forever has been bad, and this will serve as the rationale for the continued oppression of fat people.

2

. . . .

Antidotes to Medical Discourse
about Fatness

Fat has been around for ages, at varying levels of appreciation or disdain, but it has captured national attention as a public health problem in the United States during the last twenty years. Indeed, the predominant discourse about fat in Western culture today is a medical one that pathologically constructs fat bodies as "obese." "From 1960 to 1980, one quarter of U.S. adults were obese (defined as 20 percent over their desirable weight), according to the National Center for Health Statistics. Since 1980, that number has ballooned to one third of adults."[1] Since then, few periodicals are without regular, alarming articles about this public health "crisis" for which there seems to be no good reason, other than a lack of control.

Though the problem of obesity is seen by experts to have grown to national proportions, it strikes different groups within the United States with varying intensity. Likelihood of obesity varies among racial and gender groups; in a 1994 study, "while less than a third of white women and

non-Hispanic white or black men were overweight, nearly half of His-
panic or black women were."[2] According to the Technology Assessment
Conference Panel of the National Institutes of Health (NIH), the causes
of obesity are unknown. However, "evidence suggests that overweight is
multifactorial in origin, reflecting inherited, environmental, cultural, socioeconomic, and psychological conditions."[3]

Despite this conviction, obesity is popularly attributed to gluttony and
lack of exercise, both things related to the individual's lack of control.
Research at the Centers for Disease Control and Prevention "showed
58.1% of adults reporting irregular or no physical activity during leisure
time. . . . Other possible factors were cultural influences, misconceptions
or inadequate knowledge about diet, and 'a trend toward greater consumption of foods away from home.' "[4] It is not surprising, then, that
interventions to improve the health of obese individuals most often target
individual behaviors. Before I detail several of these interventions, it is
important to understand the illnesses to which obesity is alleged to have
a strong (often causal) relationship, and to explain how it has come to be
of concern to health professionals.

Researchers at the Centers for Disease Control and Prevention suggest
a connection between obesity and "higher rates of diabetes, gout, osteo-
arthritis, and other health problems."[5] Furthermore, risks of obesity include

> insulin resistance, diabetes mellitus, hypertrigliceridemia, decreased levels of
> high-density lipoprotein cholesterol, and increased levels of low-density lip-
> oprotein cholesterol. Obesity is also associated with gallbladder disease and
> some forms of cancer as well as sleep apnea, chronic hypoxia and hyper-
> capnia, and degenerative joint disease. Obesity is an independent risk factor
> for death from coronary heart disease.[6]

These illnesses have given obesity the reputation among lay people of
a dangerous, life-threatening causal agent. The obesity scare also receives
a great deal of professional attention. In 1994, a coalition including former surgeon general C. Everett Koop and the American Cancer Society
urged President Clinton to declare obesity a "national health crisis, and
to create a President's Council on Diet and Health."[7]

Based on findings that indicate that obesity increases both morbidity
and mortality risks, "it seems reasonable from a public health viewpoint
to urge all persons in the United States to maintain an average or some-

what below-average weight. Much can be gained in quality and duration of life and in reduced health costs by such a policy."[8]

A panel at the NIH Technology Assessment Conference urges "interdisciplinary research involving all types of behavioral scientists . . . to develop and evaluate prevention programs that encourage Americans to adopt healthy eating habits and lifestyles that will affect lifelong control of weight."[9] Called to action, myriad positivist researchers are doing just that in designing interventions for obesity treatment.

Among the 33 to 40 percent of adult women and 20 to 24 percent of men currently trying to lose weight, a variety of strategies are employed, with varying rates of success.[10] Interventions designed for this population include dietary change, exercise regimens, behavior modification techniques, and drug treatment. Such programs assume an effort on the part of the individual to lose weight; thus, other portions of the obese population are not reached by these interventions and remain "unhealthy."

Dietary changes, the most commonly used weight loss strategy, include everything from caloric restriction to changes in proportions of fat, proteins, and carbohydrates consumed. Programs that involve such dietary changes have documented success over the short term. Another potential strength of dietary change programs is that "participants in formal weight loss programs may reduce baseline depression and anxiety, but only if they successfully lose weight."[11]

Dietary change programs are not without their problems, however. "Weight loss at the end of relatively short-term programs can exceed 10% of initial body weight; however, there is a strong tendency to regain weight, with as much as two thirds of the weight lost regained within one year of completing the program and almost all by five years." In addition, increasing evidence suggests that "mildly to moderately overweight women who are dieting may be at risk for binge-eating without vomiting and purging."[12]

Diets may be grounded in a number of rational and normative theories. A theory of reasoned action (which assumes that "behavioral intention is the immediate determinant of behavior and that all other factors that influence behavior are mediated through intention") comes into play in diets that include significant attempts to educate about proper nutrition.[13] However, the fact that my *knowledge* that a product is bad for me changes neither my *attitude* of love for it nor my long-term *behavior* of consuming it shows the obvious inability of this theory to account for the complexity of human behavior.

Other diets may work from elements of the Health Belief Model, the troubled offspring of stimulus-response theorists. The Health Belief Model suggests that

> individuals will take action to ward off, to screen for, or to control ill-health conditions if they regard themselves as susceptible to the condition, if they believe it to have potentially serious consequences, if they believe that a course of action available to them would be beneficial in reducing either their susceptibility to or the severity of the condition, and if they believe that the anticipated barriers to (or costs of) taking the action are outweighed by its benefits.[14]

Books such as Susan Powter's *Stop the Insanity* begin by posing a list of severe *threats* to health, based on the author's personal experience, to which fat women are said to be *susceptible*. The author then lists the *benefits* (e.g., "hot-looking body," "more attractive to men," etc.) and *costs* (virtually none, of course) to taking action. Powter builds up a sense of *self-efficacy* in her readers by showing how she, a formerly fat housewife just like them, was able to lose weight, get in shape, and become a famous millionaire, too! Finally, though she claims not to be proposing a diet, Powter issues a *cue to action* by providing her newly inspired readers with a "plan" for healthy eating. Powter's simplistic book overlooks the fact that her plan won't work for all readers, especially those not in a position to act based on decisions that prioritize their own health.

Another intervention targeted at obesity shares much of the logic of interventions involving dietary changes. Just as new diets allegedly give people new ways to lose weight, improvements in nutrition labels are said to enlighten even the worst eaters, pushing them toward health and happiness. David Kessler, Commissioner of the Food and Drug Administration under Presidents George H. W. Bush and Clinton, "lost fifty pounds in 1990, which contributed to his belief that if people are given the right food information, they too will become slim, healthy, and happy."[15] Armed with his new belief, Kessler zealously pursued and enforced tougher labeling standards. Under Kessler, "the most successful portions of the . . . overhaul set standard serving sizes for comparable products and define a host of descriptors, such as 'healthy,' light, low-fat, fat-free, and cholesterol-free."[16] Other portions of his intervention recommended mandatory nutrition education in all workplaces.

In response to the move to require employers to provide information to their workers about healthy eating, cardiologist Dean Ornish says "most Americans know they should eat less fat and exercise more, they just don't do it." Rather, "people are turning to food, alcohol and other bad habits out of loneliness and despair."[17] Furthermore, "consumers, seduced by the now officially sanctioned fat-free label, figure it's okay to eat more of the fat-free foods in a single sitting."[18]

A "reasoned-action" approach to public health seems to underlie the type of intervention that highlights nutritional labeling. While it is, of course, good for consumers to have an honest idea of what they are buying and eating, it is an inappropriate way to treat obesity. "By relying on a tiny label to overcome the cultural and even physiological factors that motivate what we eat, the agency has made a costly—and fattening—mistake."[19] Improved access to information may not change human behavior in consequential ways.

A third type of intervention used with increasing frequency to combat obesity involves drug treatment. According to the NIH Technology Assessment Conference Panel, investigational drug treatment has been effective in producing weight loss in carefully controlled research programs. In particular, phenylpropanolamine, "an over-the-counter appetite suppressant approved by the Food and Drug Administration, has some efficacy in producing weight loss."[20] Many other drugs have appeared on the scene in the past several years, with varying rates of success at inducing weight loss. In addition, the recent discovery of a gene that causes obesity has led to the development of leptin, a drug known to reduce obesity in animal test populations.

Despite the obvious problems that long-term benefits of diet drugs are poorly documented and, like other over-the-counter treatments, are easily misused, my primary concern with the dangers of drug treatment of obesity lies elsewhere.[21] Though headlines touting the breakthroughs in drug treatment appear in recent newspapers, the type of interventions they represent hark back to public health approaches of the late 1800s. In this case of science at its worst, a human condition (fatness) is reduced to the workings of a pathogenic causal agent that can be obliterated with the help of chemical compounds. Most stand-alone drug therapies assume that obesity is necessarily destructive in and of itself, without ever accounting for the ways in which environmental factors interact with and shape our perceptions of the physical condition of obesity.

The preceding three interventions attempt to address the weight-related health concerns of fat people in different ways. Interventions based on dietary changes saddle overweight individuals with the historically unsuccessful task of losing weight and maintaining "normalcy" in order to be healthy. Interventions that aim to clarify food-labeling information again put responsibility for health in the hands of newly "enlightened" overweight people, who are assumed to effect dietary changes based on this newfound data. Drug treatment interventions proceed from a somewhat different angle; they locate the cause of the problem on the biological level and introduce foreign substances to the body to combat the problem that the "will" has been slow to conquer. Despite their differences, all three types of interventions share a lack of concern for the elements of the environment that have negative consequences for the health of fat people. Though some community-based approaches to weight loss and control do focus on improving such environmental factors for fat people, the main focus remains individual weight loss as a guarantor of improved health.[22] However, assertions that individual weight loss (predicated by drugs, dietary changes, etc.) saves individual lives ignore the extent to which the stigmatization of obesity is responsible for many of the health problems associated with obesity. A true intervention in the status of obese individuals in American society would make important inroads to health for even those fat people who are not actively trying to lose weight.

Angela Kennedy echoes this sentiment; in light of startling statistics that 98 percent of people who diet to lose weight will regain the weight, she muses, "No wonder health professionals cannot get job satisfaction in treating fat people. But the problem is that perhaps we are fighting the wrong enemy. By making careless assumptions about the health of fat people, we are making them ill."[23] But of course it is not the responsibility of health professionals alone to fight the outright stigmatization of fat; this political battle needs to be fought on multiple cultural fronts, with the medical field representing one of the most significant.

According to Carol Miller et al., "stereotypes about obese people . . . are pervasive, and people blame the obese for their condition."[24] As the foci of society's negative expectations, obese people face discrimination, and they have unequal access to resources, including resources that would be conducive to their health. Prejudice directed toward obese people potentially affects how they think about themselves, which has obvious disempowering health consequences.

Links to other disempowered groups abound: the prevalence of over-weight "is disproportionately high in many populations, especially in women, the poor, and members of some ethnic groups."[25] Statistics from the Centers for Disease Control that show that the highest pro-portions of overweight people are African American women (49.5%) and Mexican American women (47.9%) support Richard Klein's asser-tion that "you get fatter in this country as you get poorer, thinner as you get richer. . . . In America, money triumphs over the most resistant fat, which eventually succumbs to the regimes that only the very rich, or the fanatical, can afford."[26] Is it coincidence that representatives of these two stigmatized racial and ethnic groups, as well as women, are most likely to be obese?

An investigation of the political economy of fat suggests that the con-nection is not due to chance:

> Obesity—That ugly noun, with its inescapable pejorative implications, this term for unhealthy corpulence, has been mobilized by the medical-health-beauty establishment, and wielded by food packagers, in order to stigmatize people who do not conform to an absurdly restrictive concept of ideal weight. The image of the body beautiful, the ideal of health it promotes, is an ideological construct, a false nature, conceived by a vast industry in order to sell its services and move its products.[27]

Recognizing the restrictive meaning of "health" as proposed by weight loss programs, I would suggest that the stigma of obesity makes the most effective target for interventions that seek to improve the health status of fat Americans.

Public health interventions that target the stigmatization of obesity are fighting an uphill battle. Even at the genetic level, models of obesity are attributed to "defects" rather than a less loaded word like "variants."[28] If our fat cells start with such a bad rap, one can imagine the stigma attached to an entire *person* with an abundance of said "defects."

One suggestion, then, for fighting the power of language to create such stigma is to reform our vocabularies surrounding issues of obesity, over-weight, and health. Klein points out that *obese,* from the Latin *obesus,* meaning "having eaten well," "had a sinister rebirth in popularity . . . in the hands of nineteenth-century doctors and health workers seeking to wield power over bodies by policing the language with which one might once have referred, for example, to someone's *embonpointment.*" In a parallel fashion, *fat* has metamorphosed from a flattering term used by the Greeks, and a Teutonic root meaning "to hold or contain like a precious vessel," to its unequivocally negative connotations today.[29]

Language changes that revalue fat are among the many interventions designed and deployed by the National Association to Advance Fat Acceptance (NAAFA), a national grassroots organization devoted to improving the quality of life for fat people through public education, research, advocacy, and member support. Though the group has experienced internal conflict over whether they view fat as a normal condition or as a disability,[30] many of their strategies are healthy and empowering because they fight the stigmatization of fat instead of waging a losing battle for long-term weight reduction. They reappropriate *fat* as a term of worth and value, in an attempt to rescue it from its present pejorative status.

Unlike those who may balk at the power of discourse to alter reality, and choose instead to focus solely on material changes, NAAFA's work is aimed at highlighting the importance of community, environment, and policy—rather than searching for genetic causes or behavioral changes in the host—in the quest for health for fat people. Among their strategies are Washington-based protests for civil rights, lobbying health care professionals for tolerance and acceptance, organizing against health care/insurance discrimination, and bringing to light the political aspects of all "scientific" weight loss programs.

I will discuss one particular intervention grounded in elements of media advocacy and community organizing that had a strong impact against the stigmatization of fat, thus improving the health of fat people. The impetus for the intervention was former surgeon general C. Everett Koop's December 1994 announcement that he would launch his "Shape Up America!" program at a White House ceremony. The program was based on Koop's report "Weighing in for America's Health: Elevating Healthy Weight and Physical Fitness as a National Priority," in which fatness is named as a "multibillion dollar drain on the U.S. economy" owing to hospital care, physician services, weight reduction products and services, indirect costs of lost output, and workdays lost to illness attributable to obesity.

NAAFA organized a counter-campaign to dispel the stigmatizing idea of obesity as a public health crisis and pointed to the economics of Koop's crusade in a move supportive of Judith Butler's notion that "the very shape and form of bodies, their unifying principle, their composite parts, are always figured by a language imbued with political interests." NAAFA explained that Shape Up America! "will have $30 million in funding over the next three years [from] corporate sponsors who have each pledged $1 million, including Weight Watchers International, Campbell Soup, Heinz Foundation, . . . and the Kellogg Company."[31] Furthermore, "the program's National Advisory Committee includes obesity researchers [who] are either affiliated with weight loss programs or receive research funding from weight loss programs."[32] Whereas such organizations as the American Public Health Association joined Koop's coalition, NAAFA was able to lobby the Society for Nutrition Education (SNE) to decline. By way of explanation to Koop, SNE stated:

> SNE shares your commitment to prevention, to physical activity, and to the public's health and well-being . . . [However,] we support a new weight paradigm that opposes fat phobia, deals honestly with the difficulties of long term maintenance of weight loss, accepts the goal of health promotion and quality of life rather than slenderness, and recognizes the rights of heavy people to make decisions about their own goals and behavior.[33]

Such a refusal by a professional association reflects the inroads being made by the community organization efforts of groups like NAAFA in redefining health. In this case, Koop's ceremony was followed up by a press conference in which representatives from various size-rights organizations criticized and debunked Koop's goals and assertions. The lack of national coverage received by Koop was seen by Sally Smith, then NAAFA president, as evidence of the success of the press conference: "We succeeded in convincing reporters that this is a multi-faceted, well-funded attempt to engage Americans in another round of weight obsession, and that the underlying principles and assumptions of the program are faulty. Given the credibility and popularity of the former Surgeon General, the lack of coverage was very significant."[34]

This intervention has at its foundation principles from both community organization and media advocacy. According to Lawrence Wallack, "the mass media are effective in setting the public agenda and stimulating public discussion. The mass media confer status and legitimacy on issues and thereby make it acceptable and easier to discuss issues. . . . This power to stimulate and frame discussion is a power worth working for."[35] NAAFA's exultation over the lack of coverage given to Koop's crusade could be greater only if more coverage had been given to NAAFA's protest itself.

It is important to note that NAAFA does not use the media as a catalyst for direct changes in behavior. It assumes its audience to be agents capable of making meaning of mediated messages that, in combination with other factors, such as community discussion, may change their health behaviors or their perceptions of the role of the environment.

Instead of merely applying concepts from social marketing theory to media advocacy in the hope of increasing awareness of health issues, NAAFA advances social and political health interventions through the strategic use of mass media. "Media advocacy utilizes several important community organization concepts, including empowerment, citizen participation, and involvement in issue selection."[36]

Wallack suggests a number of essential skills, including "research, 'creative epidemiology,' issue framing, and gaining access to media outlets" to promote media advocacy.[37] Research skills involve the ability to locate important studies on obesity, mortality, and related illnesses and to be aware of any areas of contestation around obesity. NAAFA does this quite well, for example, by citing studies that show increased mortality rates among dieting women.

Creative epidemiology means framing existing research to grab the media's attention (and thus, the public's attention) and to show an issue's importance to public health. This is exactly what NAAFA did in its counterattack on Koop, by denying cause-effect relationships between obesity and related illnesses, instead presenting them as correlational.

Reframing of issues "focuses attention on industry practices, not the behavior of the individual, as the problem," resulting in "increased support for regulatory measures that can have a substantial public health impact."[38] In addition, reframing seeks to show hidden exploitative, unethical industry practices. NAAFA's effort to unveil the financial interests of corporations funding Koop's crusade calls into question the "natural" inclination to view fat as unhealthy. Indeed, it suggests that our conceptions of health are, to some extent, constructed by parties who stand to profit from them.

Finally, access to mass media outlets is very important, as airtime or space in these outlets is usually prohibitively expensive. Community members can access free media by creating "local reaction" to public health issues, by presenting small research studies, by building on related news opportunities, by providing op-ed pieces to editors.[39] NAAFA's Washington demonstration and press conference are just two instances that attracted local media attention.

Obesity is widely understood as a major health problem among Americans today, though large national organizations like NAAFA are making slow headway on this issue. However, I think that medicalized conceptions of fatness are being eroded on the micro level, as well. Everyday people negotiate their relationships to health and medical discourses using themes found in both medicalized obesity and socially constructed fatness.

3

. . . .

Sexy/Beautiful/Fat

It is difficult to extricate talk about sexuality from talk about beauty, as the two discourses fuse together like tendrils of a grapevine. However artificially, I separate the two topics into different sections here for the sake of clarity, despite my awareness that they could also be treated together. Any mainstream discussion of sexy bodies typically excludes the fat body. In this section, I examine a number of challenges to this exclusion in both "mainstream" and "alternative" media, because I believe such an exploration provides a useful backdrop to the pro-fat struggles analyzed in later chapters.[1] Obviously, the pro-fat struggles by everyday people in which I am interested do not take place in a cultural vacuum; many of the media representations of fat sexuality discussed here exert significant influence on the micro level of interpersonal communication.

The challenges that I examine first are useful inasmuch as they expose the common discursive positioning of fat people as either asexual or perverse. In media sources, challenges to conventional ways of thinking about fat sexuality (or thoughts of it *at all*) do not come often. According to Debbie Notkin, a fat woman

> is always fat, and always a woman. Traditional stereotypes of the fat woman range from the fat lady in the circus through the jolly fat aunt in the family circle to the lovely fat models of Renoir and Degas (who, although beautiful, never seem like real people). In our generation, images of fat women are frequently figures of fun, occasionally villainesses, often "bad examples" of people with no self-control or low self-esteem. Like "corporate lawyer" or "sullen teenager," the phrase "fat woman" contains the implication that you now know all you need to know about the person being discussed.[2]

In a study of print media, including books and periodicals, the vast majority of sources I encountered which discussed body image or body size presented, as Notkin predicts, *no* challenge whatsoever: fat women are depicted as ugly, disgusting, sometimes laughable objects of derision, or as pitiful victims of bad genes and psychological anomaly, whose greatest ambition is to lose fifty pounds and thereby solve all of their problems.

I had tremendous difficulty finding much work in mainstream media (e.g., articles from the dominant mainstream like *Ladies' Home Journal*, *McCall's*, *People Weekly*, and major daily newspapers, and even from the nondominant mainstream, such as *Ebony* and *Essence*) that varied from the usual declarations of "thin is in" and discussions of the wonders of this year's model diet. A sample of over three hundred articles from 1986 to 1993 that were coded for the subjects *fat* or *obesity*, or which examined the body size issues of pop icons such as Oprah Winfrey, Delta Burke, and Roseanne, revealed only fifty-five articles that seemed like potential challenges by virtue of title or title and abstract alone. After reading those fifty-five, I was able to locate only three articles that represented fat challenges (while noting the apparent insufficiency of their subversiveness).[3]

Even more difficult to obtain were challenges from "alternative" culture; this, I imagine, more accurately reflects the restricted circulation of alternative material in general than it does a lack of fat challenges from the margin. At this point, most of my alternative sources are much less accessible because of limited distribution and steep purchase prices (compare the $6 price tag on a zine for fat dykes and its Bay Area release with the international availability of a $3 glossy women's magazine). This is not to say that alternative culture is exactly brimming with resources for fat folks—yet when the margin *does* deal with body size and body image, their messages are more likely to contain challenges to traditional ways of thinking about sexual representations of fat.

Given that these challenges come in a variety of forms, it is necessary to examine the varying intensities with which they are presented. As commonly understood, a spectrum of political tendencies might be marked by assimilation at one end and by liberation at the other.[4] A fat "assimilationist" works to secure tolerance for fat rights and experiences and tries to raise consciousness about fat oppression but still possibly conceives of fat as a problem. The fat assimilationist is not unlike many disability activists who work for equal rights for an unfortunate group of handicapped people. In contrast, a fat "liberationist" celebrates fatness and tries to secure for the fat a positively valued experience of difference from the norm; she or he recognizes fat as a problem only to the unenlightened and as a boon to fat people with "abundant" experiences. The fat liberationist can be compared to disability activists who champion the beauty, potential, and unusual experiences of disabled people. Roughly arrayed, then, eight sample challenges follow, ranging from most assimilating to most liberating.

Rosemary Bray's article "Heavy Burden" appeared in *Essence* in January 1992. This autobiographical piece uses emotional description to share one African American woman's experience of fatness and dieting as a cultural outsider (i.e., a black in a white world, a fatty in a thin world, and a woman in a man's world). Bray presents a challenge in her reminder that she is still learning to "separate what is my problem and what is the world's problem" in her ordeal as a fat woman. Bray recognizes the dangers inherent in the shame that accompanies being fat when she says, "I realize now that I tolerate a level of disrespect from people about being fat that I would never, ever permit about being Black or female. It is a tolerance born of shame, an undercurrent so pervasive that I have trouble even typing the word *fat*."[5] Inasmuch as Bray refuses to offer any miracle cure and to tell her audience how to take control of their lives, her article serves to get readers thinking about the experience of being fat (rather than of trying to be thin).

Bray's article can be considered assimilating in that it concentrates on resigning fat women to the presence of a losing battle with food. She urges women to "stand watch" over this battle as she literarily talks of fat black women's oppression, then sighs and offers that to accept oneself is the passive (but never completely attainable) task at hand:

I can still be persuaded, when I'm not in my right mind, that thin people are happier, prettier, more focused, more balanced. At those moments I can still be persuaded that thin people have richer lives, that they're better people than I am. But that is the wounded me. And I am learning, at last, to love and care for her as best I can. . . . Sometimes the pain of life makes her ravenous, and I watch her eat, and I worry about both of us. And sometimes I can calm her, remove her from the fray, look after her until she is stronger. These days, the two of us are in grudging negotiation, after years and years of war with food and with each other. For today, there is no miracle.[6]

Notice Bray's dissociation of herself from the experiences (including the unmentioned pleasures) of her own body in this passage; she does little to celebrate the pleasures of fat. Instead, she assimilates by recognizing her ravenousness as a problem from which she needs to recover.

Found in another widely circulated magazine targeted to African American women and men, *Ebony*, is the next challenge, Roxanne Brown's article "Full-Figured Women Fight Back: Resistance Grows to Society's Demand for Slim Bodies." This article showcases the political and personal accomplishments of several African American women of size in resistance to society's demand for slim bodies. Brown uses the stories of successful black women to challenge tradition by presenting images of fat women in a sexually and personally appealing way, which urges readers to accept the idea that most fit bodies come in a variety of sizes. For instance, she quotes television actress Roz Ryan as saying, "I really have a thing about society deciding what we should look like. . . . If your husband feels like that [negative about your weight], get rid of him, get him out of your face. Your job is to start believing that God didn't make no mistakes."[7]

Brown's piece is assimilating in that the majority of portraits she offers of attractive fat black women are of actresses and fashion models—women whose money, glamour, and conventionally attractive faces may have earned them success *in spite of* their body sizes. For instance, references to the pretty face and youthful glow of "bubbly-natured" Madelyn Tomkins, a fat model and makeup artist, showcase Tomkins's excitement with the garment industry's recent introduction of attractive large-sized clothing rather than the pleasure she may take in her own big body. Brown takes fewer pains to celebrate fat than she does to celebrate a consumer culture in which even big fat black women can (once in a while) become moderately successful.

A significantly smaller number of people encounter the next challenge,

Rump Parliament, a bimonthly forum for discussion of size acceptance activism "to change the way society treats fat people" (cover). In that this zine's very subhead points to the "fat problem" as society's intolerance rather than the troubles caused *by* fat individuals, a challenge is immediately present. Articles in the issue back up the challenge by promoting events, such as "No Diet Day," which promote uninhibited eating.

Rump Parliament columns such as Daniel Pinkwater's "I'm Going to Say It!" proclaim the benefits of fat, despite the fact that "fat people are a maligned and oppressed minority." Claiming the upper hand on each count, Pinkwater humorously explains how his "sphericality" exempted him from participation in boring sports: "I didn't have to participate in sports, other than when I felt like it. The fact is, many fat people are good athletes, although they should not expect to excel in the track and field category."[8] His size also, to his delight, excused him from military service: "If Bill Clinton and Dan Quayle had been my size at the appropriate time, they would have had nothing to explain later. Incidentally, this is another example of retrograde thinking on the part of society at large. A human tank or land-blimp battalion would strike terror in the hearts of the enemy, and be very pleasing to view in parades." Pinkwater credits his fat body with his success as a ladies' man: "Many men dismiss me as nonthreatening because of my globularity, and therefore I get along well with competitive, A-type, killer-instinct, macho individuals—and women love me because I haven't had to develop so many of those unpleasant male traits."[9]

Rump Parliament, though, is quite assimilating in tone in that many of its articles use the fat acceptance movement as a remedy for past abuses rather than as a liberatory device.[10] Articles send the message that though fat people might rather be thin, they can be and deserve to be happy, too. I find one short story, Terry Early's "Ozark Interlude," to be particularly assimilating in its pandering to fat women's anticipated desire to be sought after by "normal" men. Early suggests that a heightened self-image for fat people, women especially, is an insufficient end compared with the ultimate goal of being wanted by "normal" people. What may have been intended as a fictional treatise on the "I'm great even though I'm fat" theme accommodates existing ideas that fat should be disregarded in a fair world.

Another challenge with limited circulation is the *NAAFA Newsletter: The Official Publication of the National Association to Advance Fat Acceptance.* As discussed in the chapter on medical discourse, NAAFA seeks to improve the lives of fat people through education, advocacy, and support. Its primary means of communication with members is through the newsletter, which represents a challenge in its broad coverage of anti-fat discrimination and public miseducation about fat. The newsletter is a forum for members to learn of ways in which their size cohorts or allies are challenging institutions. Coverage includes, for instance, reports of a march on Washington for health care for fat people and recognition of the sizable voting block constituted by fat Americans, and stories about the implementation of public education programs to change negative attitudes, which must accompany legal changes.

Though closer to the center of the political spectrum than any of the previous challenges, NAAFA's newsletter is more assimilating than it is liberatory. The primary focus of the group and of the newsletter is the promotion of tolerance for this group of "survivors." Newsletter reports protest government agencies and influential organizations that advocate measures such as weight loss surgery and yo-yo dieting or that portray fat people in a negative light. With its emphasis on struggle for mainstream political recognition and allowance, NAAFA does not celebrate fatness; it simply tries to make life in a fat body more bearable.

The intensity of the next challenge, Vanessa Feltz's "Who Says Fat Isn't Sexy?," is surprising because of its presence in *Redbook*, a widely circulated women's magazine. Feltz's "point-of-view" piece in this traditional mainstream magazine starts with the challenging declaration that "sex is like chocolate mousse: a spoonful is nice, but a vat is better. And many men agree."[11] Feltz goes so far as to frame men who do not equate fat with sexiness as women-haters, in this comparison with men who truly do enjoy women:

> Men who genuinely love women fantasize about being smothered in sofa-sized breasts and pillowed in marshmallow thighs. Pert is okay but pneumatic is heaven. Not for them the bite-size morsel. They revel in handfuls, fistfuls, and armfuls of lusty lady. Of course, millions of men don't really like women very much. They only tolerate us emaciated, depilated, and deodorized. Men who count your calories and stand over you with a stopwatch while you do sit-ups invariably claim to be doing it for your own good. Baloney! They're simply closet woman-haters—flesh-fearing, fat-baiting misogynists. They don't lust for me. The repugnance is mutual.[12]

Though I am amazed that an article incorporating such a strong and challenging stance was published in *Redbook* of all places, I suggest that Feltz's piece not be immediately canonized as a fat liberationist text.

Besides her problematic reliance on male reaction as the ultimate litmus test of fat women's sexual subjectivity, Feltz also includes in her article a description of her self-proclaimed unattractive physical appearance. Though Feltz suggests that "the secret of sex appeal is simply liking sex," rather than looking hot, why is she so quick to dismiss the possibility that her fat body be celebrated?[13] Instead, Feltz toes the party line of acceptable physical sexuality in her statement, "I'm drop dead gorgeous above the lips and below the knees, and you'd be jealous of my shapely elbows and wrists. But the rest is billowing mush."[14] Fat liberationists would ask Feltz why the "billowing mush" is not also celebrated as beauty.

The next challenge more generously evaluates this so-called mush. Laurie Edison's and Debbie Notkin's *Women En Large: Images of Fat Nudes* is an overtly political book of nude portraiture which contains forty-one photographs of fat women, as well as an excellent section on "enlarging" politics and society through recognition and appreciation of an often strangely invisible form.

This book presents a challenge because it is visually confrontational; while it is often easy enough *not* to conjure up the images presented in words in written works, this text commands that the reader see (or at least *look at*) the images it presents. Stunning black-and-white images of big, sometimes disabled, European American, African American, and Asian American women, taken in their own homes or in comfortable places, celebrate the beauty of fat.

The written text that accompanies the photographs is aimed at exposing and destroying what Notkin claims are "the bonds of oppression and shared self-hatred" which plague fat women in a society where fat women are rarely seen, let alone seen as beautiful.[15] The text presents a challenge by creating a space for the sexual expression and appreciation of fat women. Notkin writes of women learning to appreciate their fat bodies: "Buck the trend all the way and think of your fat—not only you despite your fat, but *your fat*—as beautiful. You'll probably find demons coming at you from every corner of your mind, your history, and your socialization, explaining to you just how wrong you are."[16] She goes on to expose the fickle character of this "trend" (the subversion of which she recommends):

One of our most pervasive cultural myths is that beauty and sexuality are somehow inextricably entwined, that if you are not beautiful (by the arbitrary standards set from outside), the whole universe of sexual expression and sexual fulfillment will always be a closed book to you. Fat women battle issues of sexual attractiveness every day, from the comments our dates get in public to the pitying looks we get when out by ourselves. Some people think that fat women are easy prey; I'm told that one piece of male locker room wisdom is, "The ugly ones put out," and I've certainly read advice columns which talk about the problems of the promiscuous fat woman: "Dear, if you could only lose that weight, you wouldn't have to be so desperate."[17]

Although she recognizes the obstacles to appreciation, Notkin's text fosters positive valuation of fat women's sexuality by allowing beauty and fat to exist in the same package.

However, Notkin herself locates *Women En Large* in a politically assimilationist position, as far as *sexual* representation is concerned. She claims in a personal interview that "the book is not about sex. It's about beauty . . . and it's interesting that people automatically make the connection to sex when they see nudes." Notkin maintains that her book is targeted to fat people "who are in a place where they can even begin to think about liking their bodies"; her text is intended less to radically revamp society's perception of fat bodies than to aid fat women in feeling better about themselves. She quotes one of the models, Chupoo Alafonte, as saying that "survival is more important than acceptance"; though this seems to contradict the book's emphasis on the acceptance of fat beauty, it captures the expressed assimilationist stance of its authors, whose primary goal is to change fat women's self-perception (rather than society's perception of fat women).[18]

The next challenge, while also focused on improving the self-perception of fat women, is somewhat more directed at *enjoying* fat. Susan Stinson's *Belly Songs: In Celebration of Fat Women* is a collection of one woman's poetry, fiction, and personal essays that examine fat oppression and celebrate the beauty, strength, and sensuality of fat women. The challenge this collection represents is obvious: Fat moves beyond something we must learn to cope with to something we delight in.

In the sensuous essay "Belly Song," Stinson describes the exhilarating experience of being aware of her zaftig form while eating doughnuts in the nude:

I take my belly in my hands. It's warm. My fingers feel cool, but quickly warm, too. It has a good weight, is soft. I sit very still, and feel the pulse in my thumbs, then find the pulse in the place of my thickest fat. It's delicate and regular, there, yes, there, yes, there. It comes from the underside where my palms are resting, from the left half and the right half, from veins that curve out with the rest of me. This is not dead lard. It's my body. It's my living fat.[19]

Here, the association of fat with descriptors such as "warm," "delicate," and "living" is surely a challenge to the perception of fat as grotesque and deadly.

Other pieces of prose, such as "Magnetic Force," similarly revel in the glory of the fat body. The cultural climate names fat as a repellent force dictating that "the best that many friends and family members would wish for me is that I become thin. . . . Short of that, they wish I could live without being seen. They do their best to treat me as if I looked like someone else." But Stinson's hero is *proud* to be seen: "I am in a swimming pool with seventeen fat women. . . . Our bellies, breasts and arms press together. We lap against each other, screaming and laughing. . . . My fat spills, as always, over my bones. This force is real."[20]

Stinson's challenge is liberatory in that she recognizes the force of cultural beliefs and perceptions and still suggests the lionization of big bodies. The simple title of her poem "A Practical Guide to Successful Living," which advises fat girls to "let your shirts ride up, lie down on the cold spring dirt and get mud on your fat backs," puts a subversive devil-may-care spin on a series of actions unthinkable in a fat-hating world.[21]

If Stinson's challenge is subversive, then the last challenge of this batch is nothing shy of treasonous in its liberatory orientation. *FaT GiRL: A Zine for Fat Dykes and the Women Who Want Them* is a now-defunct Bay Area zine formerly produced by a diverse collective of fat dykes from different ethnic and class backgrounds. This thoroughly self-satisfied, often pornographic zine declares its own production to be a political act made possible by reader participation; collective members urge readers to submit "sarcastic diatribes, . . . non-linear meanderings, . . . hot sexual forays from the perverse to the sublime, . . . tales of gender play, . . . and gossip and encouragement."[22] An article in the *San Francisco Bay Times* describes the zine as full of "photos of fat girls getting it on and getting off, in various creative, nasty and sweaty ways. Here's the stuff you'll never see in *Off Our Backs!*"[23]

As it challenges even many feminist conceptions of what is acceptable or attractive, *FaT GiRL* is certainly liberatory. Photographic depictions of the shaving of a fat mons pubis, bootlicking against a backdrop of generously fleshy thighs, big naked butts, big women with tattoos and multiple body piercings enmeshed in sadomasochistic leather-and-link ensembles being fisted, and fat women erotically feeding each other forbidden foods—all this is found inside. Beyond merely celebrating their fat, the women involved with *FaT GiRL prefer* it to the bodies of their smaller sisters. Unlike other liberatory texts that fete fat to protest the hegemony of thinness, *FaT GiRL* goes so far as to exclaim that fatness is the preferred way of being in the world. An advice column called "Hey Fat Chick!" illustrates this preference in response to a worried letter from "The Invisible Blob," whose thin girlfriend gets too much attention from "thin glamour-gals":

> Girl, it's obvious you have something those catty glam-gals don't. My advice to you? *FLAUNT IT!* . . . Public Displays of Affection between the two of you can only help to remind these intrusive women that: 1) your lover is too BUSY to notice them since she is quite excited to have your tongue in her mouth, [and] 2) you obviously have something very appealing to said gf that they're missing. And by this, I mean more than a butt you can grip with both hands. *You are great and beautiful. Revel in their pathos. Feel sorry for them.*[24]

Other articles, like "Oh My God! It's Big Mama!", expose the "looksism" sometimes characteristic of lesbian communities, groups whose Othered experiences might suggest that they would know better. The author, "Barbarism," believes that both dyke and straight worlds depend on visual cues (like apparent gender, race, and body size) to define identities. She says that "when you claim your dykehood you are demanding a public sexual persona. Fat women have a sexuality? Hard bodies only. Are you height/weight proportionate?" The article unfolds an interview with a fat dyke couple, providing an opportunity to "really see" two women "in all their fat glory."[25]

Clever, angry space fillers like "Recycling Hints" also expose the liberatory orientation of *FaT GiRL*. A recipe for recycling glass Christmas ornaments finds readers pulling paint-filled bulbs from the pockets of their housedresses and aiming at anti-fat billboards and diet centers as they ride by on their motorcycles or red Schwinns with big flowered baskets at 3 A.M.[26] Pride and the reclamation of hegemonic tropes are central resignificatory strategies.

Still, even many of these so-called challenges leave the dominant ideology comfortably intact. Pieces like Bray's, which paint fat as something sexually undesirable that we must learn to live with, or even like Feltz's, which describe fat as sexually unattractive, reach large numbers of women because of their presence in widely circulated, inexpensive magazines. Though they make the important first step of questioning what the world thinks of them, both authors capitulate to the idea that fat sexuality is problematic. As I later suggest, conversations in everyday life are marked by the same kinds of contradiction, striking a balance between what they celebrate and what they dismiss, always highly contested.

Though, as I discussed in the section on historical interpretations of fatness, it certainly has not always been the case, one of the ways the fat body (especially the fat *female* body) has been constructed in the last thirty years is as an ugly body. Following structuralist thought, however, I have peppered this book with suggestions about the usefulness of such an ugly construction. Structuralists might believe that even the most pernicious challenges to traditional beauty standards, like *FaT GiRL,* are defanged by their location within a system of aesthetic ideals and beauty standards based on an innocence of the uses of knowledge and power. Despite the best emancipatory intentions, all images are contained within a timeless, universal, natural, and *impenetrable* veneer of beauty.

This perspective is criticized because it grants too much power to the alleged monolith of beauty discourse. A structuralist perspective on fat politics is unable to explain the historical changes in perceptions of fat beauty; it also ignores cultural variations of body size preference. It is too quick to reduce the fat sexual subjectivity constructed in these challenging representations to what Michael Huspek, in a different context, calls "a mere arbitrary sign bound up within a power infused system of signs."[27]

I believe that most of us view *beauty* as pure, natural, and innocent—and that *this* view not only denies the social construction of beauty but goes beyond to vanquish the objects of beauty to a strangely exclusive realm. Consider Wendy Chapkis's admonition: "However much the particulars of the beauty package may change, the basic principles remain—the borders of beauty are well defined and exceedingly narrow."[28] Fat, when celebrated by fat liberationists, is made just as innocent, just as beautiful as thin—made just as dangerous, and just as ridiculous. A post-modern perspective on the body applauds this creation and constant re-creation of fat, beautiful images that pull beauty down from its pedestal, making it accessible and omnipresent. Simply trying to liberate fat from ugliness to beauty, without questioning the paradigm of beauty itself, is quite dangerous; Butler warns about the appearance of a "liberated" body "posing as subversive but operating in the service of . . . law's self-amplification and proliferation."[29]

According to Chapkis, women's pursuit of beauty is marked by the desire for an unattainable control over identity, which causes the body to continually become Other until it finally disappears; this is problematic, she claims, especially for creatures whose existence is often reduced to a mere bodily reality. Chapkis points to the aforementioned narrowness of beauty when she says that

> for a woman, then, her traditional—if entirely unreliable—ticket to success in life and transcendence beyond it is the mortal body. The woman who is awarded the title of Beauty momentarily escapes into the eternal ideal. Yet she knows, as each woman must, that she has been or will be seen as ugly in her lifetime. To be beautiful is to exist in a moment framed by expectation and fear.[30]

For fat women, then, the goal of inclusion in such a shaky enterprise as timeless (but fragile) beauty seems questionable at first. The history of beauty, with its claims to timelessness and constancy is, according to Chapkis, deeply embedded in Western culture, from the time of the Platonic tradition. I assert, following Chapkis, that beauty's clever trick of making *itself* not seem a social construction is what makes beauty virtually impossible, at this point, to forsake.[31] Given this tradition, it is improbable that the idea of beauty will be abandoned completely. The alternative, then, is to try to redefine beauty in its own very intimidating and self-proclaimedly inert face—to proliferate the meanings of beauty so that the power of its original concept is weakened.

Chapkis maintains that "approximating beauty can be essential to a woman's chances for power, respect, and attention. Recognizing this, women have quite sensibly directed great energy toward evaluating . . . their appearance."[32] Such energy can even be conceived of as the liberatory push to celebrate fat women as beautiful not just in personality, but in appearance and sexuality, too.

On the assumption that staking a new subjectivity within the discourse of beauty is the key to empowerment for fat women, I turn to Susan Bordo's work on postmodern subjects as the foundation for envisioning a subjectivity for fat women. Bordo claims that our bodies "have become alienated products, texts of our own creative making, from which we maintain a strange and ironic detachment."[33] I see this turn less as strange and more as an opportunity; following Bordo, one might assume that the "nature" of fat women's bodies is alienated, forgotten—they are no longer trying to discover their innocent bodies as beautiful in a postmodern world. Fat bodies are sites for creation and contexts of resistance that are mediated by language; fat cannot be beauty, because beauty is purity/ innocence in a time when Bordo claims "we . . . have no direct, innocent, or unconstructed knowledge of our bodies."[34] The problem, then, with most fat assimilationists and liberationists alike within the context of beauty lies in their emphasis on tolerating or even loving themselves as beautiful *the way they are*, instead of recognizing the constructed nature of that very being.

Some of the more radical challenges from the fat liberation front do seem to recognize this constructedness and play with reinventing themselves outside the discourse of beauty (e.g., *FaT GiRL*). This type of challenge, following Bordo, attempts to "fabricate . . . through imitation and gradual command of public, cultural idioms" a new authenticity for fat women.[35] I would shift emphasis here from imitation (which is reminiscent of representing an original, a truth) to *fabrication*, the idea of making up something in order to belie some truth, which relates to *simulation*, a pretense, a feigning. The body, according to Bordo, does not exist as an out-there a priori entity; instead, it is a text within the foundation of discourse. I suggest that the fabrication or simulation of a new existence for fat women would expose the use of this text as a coercive instrument of power; it would potentially reveal that the body is never just beautiful, never innocently known, it is never immune to layerings of power/ knowledge.

If I follow Bordo's understanding of Michel Foucault, I can state that the act of flaunted fat in simulations of beauty still cannot be deemed resistant without examining its practical, historical, and institutional reverberations. For its strides in positing fat women as sexually heroic, *FaT GiRL* (as well as some of the other fat-positive discursive sites examined later) can be considered a simulation of beauty. Reminders such as the following radically rethink the boundaries of attractiveness: "Remember the last time your great belly shook with the thunderous roar of an orgasm. *Who helped you* get rid of that brainwashing bullshit about fat women having no sexuality? . . . *Fat Girl*, that's who. Yeah, she's a superhero, but she's not just one, and she doesn't fit into a fucking phone booth. She lives inside every one of us."[36]

Still, one cannot simply look at a zine like *FaT GiRL*, or a completely pro-fat on-line exchange, and say "Yes! That's it! A change-provoking resistant simulation of fat women!" because one can't stop at the textual surface of the body. Bordo believes that "subversion of cultural assumptions . . . is not something that happens *in* a text or *to* a text. It is an event that takes place (or doesn't) in the reading of a text."[37] I would argue that the same would hold for fat challenges: only an exploration of their readings would begin to explain what they really *do* to culture. While this is a necessary next step in understanding and actualizing the empowerment of fat women, one cannot deny that the "first step" of reinvention of one's fat self in an effort to alter the discourse of beauty is a highly political act with subversive cultural consequence.

4

. . . .

Citizen Profane: Consumerism, Class, Race, and Body

Anti-fat sentiment did not fall from the sky, nor is it the overdetermined product of a zealous media complex alone. Anti-fat sentiment is a by-product of the desire to be slim, which "must be understood in terms of a confluence of movements in the sciences and in dance, in home economics and political economy, in medical technology and food marketing, in evangelical religion and life insurance."[1] It manifests itself when an individual who is insecure about his or her body responds defensively "whenever he [or she] is confronted by other bodies that, by their dissimilarity, suggest the possibility that his [or her] own body could potentially and in some strangely uncontrolled way be changed or transformed."[2] People who inhabit "dissimilar" bodies are read as both inferior and threatening: inferior in terms of beauty, and threatening in terms of the suggestion of downward mobility. Fatness, with its omnipresent visual suggestion of body instability, frequently garners rejection and becomes the dubious beneficiary of legal, political, and material inequalities that are legitimated by the determining power of the biological body rather than contingent and reversible social constructions.[3] When biology is mistaken for destiny, inequalities prosper, albeit under false pretenses.

Anti-fat bias is more pronounced in individualist cultures that emphasize personal freedom and autonomous goal achievement (like the United States, Australia, or Poland) than in collectivist ones (like Mexico, Turkey, or Venezuela).[4] People's beliefs about whether or not fat can be controlled (and thus whether or not a fat person warrants insult) are linked to their more fundamental social ideologies. The endorsement of a Protestant ethic ideology leads one to view stigmatized peoples as willful violators of traditional American values such as moral character, hard work, and self-discipline.[5]

Those who argue on behalf of anti-fat bias proclaim that "social stigmas—even unfair ones—can be useful, even necessary." They argue that the impulse to legally prevent anti-fat discrimination ends in a most dystopian state: "By the time you've finished preventing discrimination against the ugly, the short, the skinny, the bald, the knobbly-kneed, the flat-chested and the stupid, you're living in a totalitarian state."[6] Slippery-slope logical fallacy notwithstanding, it is telling that stigmas are embraced as a useful means of framing notions of citizenship.

Critics flag fatness as a plague on the house of American citizenship. Questions of fit in our capitalist economy emerge, suggesting that to be fat is to fail to do one's duty as a productive worker: "Already the U.S. economy loses $100 billion from weight-related sickness . . . what chance has America in the long run, if [fat acceptance prevails], that it can ever compete with those wiry Filipinos and Koreans?"[7] This xenophobic daydream posits an unproven causal relationship between somatotype and productivity among workers. Studies completed as long ago as 1974 suggest that such claims, inasmuch as they concern mild and moderate obesity, are significantly overrated;[8] nonetheless, the attitude toward fatness as a failure of citizenship prevails. But more interesting than the *accuracy* of this claim is the intensity with which it signals a failure on the part of the fat body to register as a fully productive body in a capitalist economy.

Body type, citizenship, and moral type have been long linked: "beautiful" and "healthy" cluster to connote a "good" citizen, while "ill" and "ugly" put one in the citizenship doghouse. "The good citizen cannot be ugly and therefore cannot be infected by, or infect, members of society with dangerous illnesses, illnesses that would be marked on their physiognomies."[9] For the better part of the twentieth century, fatness was both pathologized and considered aesthetically unappealing, damning its bearers to dwell in the shadows of citizen life.

The fat person makes the ultimate bad citizen in that she or he reveals the American Dream for what it is: a fabrication. If we put stock in a philosophy of limitless individual achievement through hard work and intelligence, then what is a fat person but a sign that we can't always get what we want?[10] Because they rain on society's parade, fat people are punished. In contrast, bulimics, inasmuch as they "satisfy the insatiable needs of the capitalist machine and at the same time pleas[e] the thin-obsessed society," are the perfect citizens.[11] Only by consistently frustrating our desires can ever-increasing consumption be propelled by late capitalism. It is fat folk who suffer a bad rap, however, in the global economy; their insatiable appetites are said to divert food from where it's needed most. Some critics, though, point out the contrary idea that "thin people are capitalism's ideal consumers, for they can devour without seeming gluttonous; they have morality on their side."[12]

National governments have historically become concerned with bodies during times of social change and economic/military crisis. "Fears were expressed in the United States and Britain during the nineteenth century about overindulgence and fatness among the rich, and malnutrition among the poor. Both these issues were related to worries about racial degeneration and the degenerating stock of society."[13] Later on, during World War II, fatness was a nearly treasonable condition, not just because of perceived gluttony but because of the subsequent waste of energy. Decadent food intake without sufficient patriotic energy output was a wartime no-no.[14]

American concerns about racial and social-class purity were not, however, cast aside along with combat boots and dog tags at the end of the war. If fat people are understood as antithetical to the efficiency and productivity required to succeed in our capitalist economy, then their presence haunts as the specter of downward mobility.[15] Big, profusely round bodies also provoke racist anxieties in the white modern West because of their imagined resemblance to those of maligned ethnic and racial Others; fatness haunts as the specter of disintegrating physical privilege in this case.

Outside of the activist challenges documented elsewhere in this book, opportunities for fat people to resuscitate themselves as citizens are limited; they necessitate being subsumed by capitalist culture. Fat oppression and capitalist culture are emphatically linked, according to Nomy Lamm, whose zine *I'm So Fucking Beautiful* was a boon to fat activists in the 1990s. Lamm contends that capitalist culture "keeps us relegated to the role of pathetically needy consumer base, forever in search of the miracle diet that will change our lives."[16] A fat person's only shot at citizenship comes if he or she gratefully consumes the panoply of diet and fitness products made available by industry and government.

Within the context of a consumer market economy, female bodies are differentiated from each other simply to augment market potential.[17] Fatness is an especially important signifier in this process of demarcation. TV talk shows are one arena in which fat bodies are displayed as freakish and punished for transgressing body norms. Instead of such shows signifying a wider range of healthy body alternatives for women, the disgust enacted by both hosts and in-studio audience members cues us to read their performances negatively. Given that diet products are the top advertisers during these programs, "it is not surprising that alternative readings that embrace a variety of body types are not explored. . . . These shows engender a very specific anxiety about women's bodies in order to sell products."[18]

Even work that contains an implicit critique of capitalist consumerism still oozes anti-fat sentiment. In their 1979 book *The Overeaters,* Jonathan Wise and Susan Kierr Wise argue that "since many obese people have had trouble in early stages of ego development, their resulting immature personalities require immediate gratification. The obese have difficulty postponing their rewards and seek comfort from whatever is most easily attainable."[19] Though the critique of our postcapitalist instant-gratification lifestyle has resonance, the corresponding charges of the immaturity of fat people are unfounded and smack of similar claims made about racial and ethnic minorities.[20]

The Wises suggest that low self-esteem is common among the overweight because of our cultural preference for thinness. Troublingly, their solution to this predicament is to disentangle food from emotional development rather than to explore the viciously arbitrary nature of our cultural preferences. Dance movement therapy (admittedly, a nice break from dieting, but still done primarily for weight loss) and increased sensitivity to food are purported to save the day: "Knowing what one's hungers and needs really are and responding to internal instead of external cues are imperative for sanely balanced eating in a culture that offers immoderate amounts of consumerism—often in the form of food."[21] While the attention to the ill effects of consumerism is warranted, it need not be accompanied by the virulence of anti-fat rhetoric. Fat continues to be thoroughly reviled precisely *so that* the plethora of diet/health/fitness industry products will continue to have a reliable market base.[22]

Failures of production and consumption are not the only perceived shortcomings of the fat body, however. Fatness also marks one as a failure at attaining citizenship in the dominant socioeconomic class. In wealthy nations like the United States, social constraints against "vulgar" fatness are deployed by the dominant classes, who are "more willing and most able to produce the bodily forms of highest value, as their formation requires investments of spare time and money."[23] Today, the socioeconomically advantaged are the only ones with enough time free from the ravages of wage labor and enough money to invest in personal trainers and pricey gym memberships to be able to cultivate the corps du jour—toned and supple, with a dangerously low percentage of body fat.

In discussing just how the primped upper-class body has come to signify superiority, Pierre Bordieu suggests that the more cultured bodies are those that are furthest from nature. "The legitimate use of the body is spontaneously perceived as an index of moral uprightness, so that its opposite, a 'natural' body, is seen as an index of *laisser-aller* ('letting oneself go'), a culpable surrender to facility."[24] But just because a particular group or class manages to win most-favored-body status does not guarantee that it will continue to be so valued indefinitely. "The value attached to particular bodies changes over time; as fields within societies change, so may the forms of physical capital they reward."[25]

The vehemence with which those who enforce notions of "normality" seek to eradicate fatness is disturbing, especially for its class implications. Leslie Fiedler contends that the wealthy can always buy normality with surgery, chemicals, hormones, and the like—so when all who are capable of doing so have made themselves "homogenously, monotonously beautiful," the poor will be our last freaks.[26] As aesthetic variability fades, it is replaced by "a Grade-A, U.S.-inspected, homogenized form of pre-packaged, commercialized 'beauty.' Automation, urbanization, and mass affluence help the trend along, since these are processes that encourage a standardized physical appearance."[27]

Fatness marks the individual as a failed citizen in a number of ways: as not of the dominant social class, as an inadequate worker and consumer. But fatness seems further to render its inhabitant not racially adequate, in that anti-fat bias shares some disturbing characteristics with eugenics movements. Anti-black attitudes overlap with anti-fat bias in persons who believe that both blacks and fat people deserve their fate, and that their social and economic status is a result of circumstances that they could control.[28] The difference, however, is that there's little in the way of public norms to keep people from expressing anti-fat sentiment in public.

A November 2000 *New York Times* article on culture and obesity trumpets the predicament of white weight gainers who find themselves suddenly keeping company with black and Latino folks. " 'Obesity has been seen as a minority issue for some time, and all of a sudden minorities have company from the general population,' said Dr. Shiriki K. Kumanyika, a professor of epidemiology at the University of Pennsylvania in Philadelphia. 'This newfound attention to the problem can only benefit us all.' "[29] Though the "problem" Kumanyika refers to is likely the obesity, it is also possible to understand "the problem" as the adoption by the general (read: white) population of the kind of adipose tissue formerly held chiefly by unpreferred (black and Latino) minority groups. One might interpret the reinvigorated efforts to wipe out obesity as a sort of modern-day eugenics campaign: keep us pure by keeping us free of the "maladies" experienced by cultural Others. Alarmingly, a survey of married couples revealed that 11 percent would abort a child known in advance to be genetically predisposed to obesity.[30]

Within fat acceptance circles, this notion of eugenics carries some credence. Creative writer Donna Allegra, who is African American, declares that "white women are kept in line by racist devices as well—their beauty measured by how much they don't look like people of color. We are said to wear the characteristics, like weight on a woman's body, that are deemed unacceptable by white American beauty standards."[31] The racist power of internalized fat-phobia is a surefire tool to keep white bodies "pure" in shape and size.

Despite mainstream stigmatization of fat bodies, numerous studies done in the last twenty years suggest that African American girls are more content with their body weight and are less likely to diet than are white or Latino girls.[32] Mimi Nichter's work posits that while 15 percent of "normal"-weight black girls were dissatisfied with their weight, 90 percent of "normal"-weight white girls were. However, dieting practices were similar among blacks and whites.[33] Black girls reported personality traits—such as style, creativity, resourcefulness—as important in an ideal girl, while white girls focused more on looks.[34] These findings seem promising of resistance to an environment marked by rising incidences of eating disorders and anti-fat bias.

Another anecdote from halfway around the world supports the disparity in body-size obsession between blacks and whites. In December 2000, the *New York Times* reported on the mission to abolish obesity in South Africa, a country with more HIV-positive residents than any other worldwide. Dr. Thandi Puoane faced a stumbling block in her mission when she discovered that nearly all of the health workers at a clinic south of Cape Town were obese, "hardly the sort of models to preach the message that heavy is not healthy. And worse, most of the workers were not the least bit worried about their weight."[35] The *Times* is correct; these health workers would make horrible fat teetotalers, because they are thriving in a health-hostile environment. The righteousness inherent in suggesting that there is something wrong with these workers feeling no shame about their fatness is distinctly American and Western European. When one of the health workers is quoted as saying, "If you are overweight you don't look nice," after a health-reeducation session, I cannot help but hear the line in a spaced-out, Stepford Wives type of intonation: "Yes, master, I look bad and feel bad. Yes."[36] One of the chief reasons for reluctance to lose weight there is that thinness is conceptually linked to the ravages of HIV in South African communities . . . but what is most important to those trained in Western medicine is to inculcate shame about one's body as a means of promoting "health."

Unsurprisingly, similar self-smearing anti-fat campaigns thrive in the United States, too, and are even supported by the federal government. Apparently, the National Institutes of Health finds some African American women's positive attitude toward healthy, full-figured bodies rather troubling. A report of the National Heart, Lung and Blood Institute (NHLBI) concludes that "such an assumption may be a barrier in attempting to work with overweight African American women who—although they may want to weigh less and be healthier—do not necessarily consider themselves unattractive or overweight, and may value cosmetic aspects of body weight less."[37] It seems that the NHLBI would prefer a degraded sense of self-esteem among black women, in that they would be more likely to diet out of aesthetic desperation that way. What are we to do with black women who feel good about themselves? Medical establishments far and wide would prefer to convince them that they are deluded—a convenient move for ensuring their dependence on the medical industry.

Statistics like those presented by Nichter, and anecdotes about defiantly fat South African health care workers, have an unfortunate effect, however, inasmuch as they propel a fetishizing of black attitudes about fat bodies. T. J. Bryan points out the problem in white women putting black/African fat acceptance on a pedestal:

> My Noble Savage (N.S.) triggers are coming fast and furious. Supposedly the last planetary receptacle of primitive spirituality, aesthetics and culture not tainted by the effects of white western civilization. Artistic and intellectual property, a legacy . . . now also serves as a mirror, a tool. Reflecting not him/herself but the beauty, insecurities and body issues of Western/non-Black/non-African heavy wimmin, instead. I am frustrated by the unspoken power inherent in the assumption of one hegemonic fatty girl voice.[38]

When research on views of fatness in black communities actually includes the voices of black individuals, fatness tends to be described as a contradictory and discrimination-prompting state, rather than as some utopic mode of being. Furthermore, "the discrimination against [fat black women] is so faceted that the society often confuses their fatness with their poverty and both with ignorance. To say in their defense that blacks like fat or that poor people appreciate a bit of extra weight is a forbiddingly neat way to cut them off from the rest of society, to limit their economic and social range."[39]

Other critics argue that fat acceptance in African American communities is a myth. Regina Williams, chair of the Detroit chapter of NAAFA, believes that acceptance is forthcoming for women with large breasts or buttocks but says "Don't let us get *too* big or we're classified as undesirable."[40] (It should be noted, though, that while women sized 16–22 are considered full-figured and desirable in African American communities, according to Williams, women of the same sizes are considered fat and undesirable in white middle-class communities.) Williams acknowledges that African American assimilation attempts have resulted in their adoption of a Eurocentric beauty standard. Indeed, so-called upward mobility, whether from a nonwhite racial base or from a working-class socioeconomic base, typically involves the embrace of a thinner body ideal.

Media aimed at African American communities are increasingly re-

minding black folk to pursue slenderness as heartily as their white peers
do. Experts on African American obesity are trotted out with increasing
frequency to attest to the fact that obesity rates for young black people
have more than doubled in the past twenty years and to certify that white
teen girls are 60 percent less likely to be overweight than black teen girls.[41]
A January 2001 *Essence* article told the triumphant tale of young Alexa
Andrew, who lost twenty pounds after learning she had diabetes: "It's
amazing how well she's done,' says her mother. 'She lost more than 20
pounds, is willing to get into a bathing suit to go swimming and now
enjoys shopping for clothes!' Alexa's self-esteem had also suffered because
of her weight, but now she's as vain as most adolescents. 'She lives in the
mirror, and you can't tell her anything,' says Janice [her mother]."[42]

It seems an odd move to applaud the self-absorption that vanity entails.
That this is taken as a sign of progress verifies the hegemony of white
beauty standards. However, a counter-discourse circulates within these
same media, reminding black readers that fat is seen as healthy in their
communities and that fleshier bodies, rather than stick figures, are preferred by black men[43]—a conclusion that begs feminist deconstruction for
its overreliance on male sanctification of female bodies.

Parallels in Afro-Caribbean culture indicate a similar regard for fatness.
In her study of body image in rural Jamaica, ethnographer Elisa Sobo
affirms that "amassing wealth and keeping slim have antisocial connotations." Communal money and food means nobody gets too rich or too
thin. While they value large size, some Jamaicans differentiate between
"good" and "bad" fat, "the good being firm like a fit mango and the bad
being spongy, soft, hanging slack, and denoting declining fitness as if a
person was an overripe fruit, beginning to break down or rot."[44] Again,
we see that fatness is endorsed only to a certain degree, and not embraced
without exception, as is the goal of many fat activists. On the whole,
though, it is easy to see that fatness is perceived to be aligned with black
and Latino racial minorities and is thus undesirable for the righteous
(white) citizen.

Though fatness has most recently indicated a failure of citizenship, it
doesn't always have to carry out this same function. It is true that "the
possibility of passing, trying to lose weight, wanting to become 'normal',
is about the only recognized option available to fat women in twentieth-
century Anglo-American culture."[45] However, the theorist Chris Shilling
argues that this type of phenomenon is a result of our (changeable) ten-

dency in the affluent West to see the body as something in the process of becoming; it is "a *project* which should be worked at and accomplished as part of an *individual's* self-identity."[46] While he discusses health, plastic surgery, and bodybuilding as examples of this drive, one could certainly consider fat activism a body project of another sort. Perhaps, though, fat activism entails a process of giving up the idea that the body itself is a project, instead replacing it with the project of resuscitating the body's citizenship. Cultural historian Hillel Schwartz reminisces about fat utopias, like Servia, Indiana, circa 1899, or Roseto, Pennsylvania, in the 1960s, where fat people, because they were the norm, were free from the need to regard their bodies as projects. In a fat utopia, Schwartz imagines, "fat women would not live in the future conditional, suspended between what they are and who they will be when they are finally thin."[47] Getting to this point means recognizing that "fat, like beauty and appearance, can be read in a political context; the stigma attached to being fat is a control mechanism which supports a power structure of one group of people over another, and fat politics is a way of challenging that status quo."[48]

I close this chapter with an example that illustrates how the stigma of fat clusters around the stigma of poverty and of nonwhiteness with the effect of depriving individuals of their rights as citizens. Widely publicized cases of fat children removed from their homes—their bodies taken as evidence of their abuse and neglect at the hands of their parents—typically involve people of color and the poor or working class. The case of New Mexico resident Anamarie Regino, a 130-pound three year old, is worthy of an analysis that considers the role of her family's underdog status (Mexican American ethnicity and working-class rank) in the decision to remedy Regino's fatness by ripping the family apart. Adela Martinez-Regino, Anamarie's mother, explained that despite her native-language English fluency, the social worker insisted on speaking to her in Spanish. She claimed, "Something this important, I want to understand everything, and her English was perfect. But she decided that mine wasn't. She decided all sorts of things. She kept asking for phone numbers of my family in Mexico. I kept telling her I was born and raised here. My mother was born here. She wanted us to be ignorant foreigners so she could write that in her report."[49] The social worker's affidavit, which recommended foster care for Anamarie, concluded by stating that "the family does not fully understand the threat to their daughter's safety and welfare due to language or cultural barriers."[50] Eventually, Anamarie was returned to her home amidst a whirl of suspicions that her family was still abusing her through overfeeding; an anonymous informant tipped off Children, Youth and Family Services that she had been seen in public eating ice cream. Her attorney, Troy Prichard, suggested that the surveillance of Ana resonated with an attitude of "You know those Mexican people, all they eat is fried junk, of course they're slipping her food."[51]

The Regino case illustrates how anti-fat bias is often rife with racist and classist presuppositions. Inherent in the state's motion to remove Ana from her home are the beliefs, first, that to be obese is to be abused and, second, that people from certain "low-rent" groups—in this case, working-class Mexican Americans—are culpable in the abuse because of a combination of unacceptable cultural traditions and ignorance. Anamarie Regino and those like her—failed consumers, ethnic Others, the working poor—flunk their citizenship tests, rendering them the citizens profane of contemporary American culture.

5

. . . .

Revolution on a Rack: Fatness, Fashion, and Commodification

Fat offends Western ideals of female beauty and, as such, every "overweight" woman creates a crack in the popular culture's ability to make us mere products.

SUSIE ORBACH, *Fat Is a Feminist Issue*

Commodification is the mode through which contemporary Western societies seek to ensure a minimal continuity in how people present themselves. That is, the means for managing the self have become increasingly tied up with consumer goods, and the achievement of social and economic success hinges crucially on the presentation of an acceptable self-image.

CHRIS SHILLING, *The Body and Social Theory*

Manufacturers and retailers have realized that, demographically in age and income, full-figured women are identical to their thinner counterparts.

ERIKA D. PETERMAN, "A Big Idea Catches On"

In 1997, on a visit to New York City, I wander into The Body Shop, where an enormous poster greets me. A sassy red-headed doll resembling Barbie's fat cousin reclines on a green brocade divan, her full, pendulous breasts gently sloping toward her spare-tire waist. The large caption reads, "There are 3 billion women who don't look like supermodels and only 8 who do." In smaller print, the poster commands its reader: "Love your body." I am stunned at the audacity of the image and text; why is a cosmetics company, which sells its customers hope in a jar, telling me that "self-esteem is truly the route to revolution"?[1] What motivates this bastion of popular culture to license me to appreciate my own body, instead of comparing it (unfavorably) to others?

A year later, while channel surfing, I come across the Emmys just in time to catch Camryn Manheim, star of *The Practice* and bodacious fat chick, beaming during her edgy acceptance speech, and declaring of her award: "This is for all the fat girls!"[2] Is this public acknowledgment, appreciation even, of fat women? This moment of celebration trumps decades of "diet or die" mentality in Hollywood.

I chart this brief trajectory of experiences and observations in order to understand how the fat body morphed from an egregious aesthetic affront into the commodifiable aesthetic entity it is today. Paralleling Danae Clark's work on commodity lesbianism, I want to examine the relationship between fat women and consumer culture, representations of fat women and consumption in media texts, and the role of the fat woman spectator as a consuming subject.[3]

There are a number of reasons for advertisers' historical apathy toward fat women. Studies suggest a definitive link between socioeconomic class and obesity, with obesity "six times more common among women of low status as compared to those of high status."[4] Thus, fat women have been perceived to lack purchasing power, despite the fact that fatness does exist among the wealthy. Furthermore, fat women cross age, race, as well as income boundaries, and thus present an unfocused target for advertiser efforts. Finally, advertisers may want to avoid the association of their products with the stigma of fatness, as negative connotations have the power to undo a company. Indeed, Argentinian legislator Maria del Carmen Banzas states that "the fashionable brand names that target adolescents do not want 'chubby' girls using their clothing, because they believe that would hurt their brand name, which is identified with languid, anorexic models."[5]

Fat women have not, until recently, been targeted with any zeal as a particular customer group. For many years, the fat woman was indeed the forgotten woman, invisible in advertising and strictly limited to comic or tragic roles in fictional media depictions.[6] In the late 1990s, though, fat women have emerged as all-too-eager consumers. While growth in retail clothing sales is essentially flat, plus-size segment growth ranks at 10 to 11 percent annually and has shown consistent increases.[7] David Defeo, president of a plus-size clothing manufacturing company, explains that focus group research "found that women were very frustrated by the shopping experience they were getting and by the assortment in stores."[8] Roz Pactor, a fashion executive at Foley's, a Denver store, says that retailers now realize that "these women are hungry for fashion, they've got money to spend, and if they like it, they'll buy it. All that was offered for years was dumb styling. Now there are all these great resources."[9]

Though the precise impetus for the commodification of corpulence is unclear, it may be owed in part to the relatively new perception that fat consumers now have considerable disposable income. *Mode* magazine cofounder Nancy LeWinter asserts that "manufacturers and retailers have realized that, demographically in age and income, full-figured women are identical to their thinner counterparts."[10] Sometimes government concerns provoke commodification: in 2000, the Argentine Senate debated a bill to mandate the production of a larger range of sizes for women by garment manufacturers, "to keep from marginalizing a sector of consumers and avoid contributing to the emergence of eating disorders."[11] Whatever the reason, fat women are now both self-identified as and hailed by capitalist enterprise as consumers.

Long ghettoized in specialty stores, fashions for "plus-size" girls are now becoming mainstreamed. Girlfriends, a California-based clothing catalog, operates with the tagline "fashion and fit for all sizes."[12] Sizes on most items range from 0 to 25, or XS through 3XL, and among the regularly used fresh-faced teen models is an attractive, broadly smiling fat girl. And she doesn't wear a muu-muu, either; instead, she sports the clingy "boyfriend tank" and shiny "zuma board shorts," just like her peers. Although her one-piece bathing suit is arguably more staid than the triangle-top bikini shown off by a more slender girl, it's in the same loud pattern and bright colors as everyone else's suit.

Lane Bryant is another company that has capitalized tremendously on fat women's enthusiastic consumer impulses after recovering from a stale fashion– and poor management–induced slump in the early nineties.[13] Until 1998, the business received criticism from fat women for advertisements that featured only the usual willowy-framed models. However, when they began featuring celebrities like Manheim, Kathy Najimy, Anna Nicole Smith, and Queen Latifah, they began to appeal to potential customers who, for the first time, recognized their image (or one at least in the same species) in the public eye. One of Lane Bryant's most recent advertising maneuvers involves the depiction of actor Chris Noth, who plays "Mr. Big" on HBO's *Sex and the City,* cozying up with conventionally beautiful, plus-sized models. Marketing executive Chris Hansen acknowledges that the portrayal of a man endorsing and enjoying fat women's bodies in a sexual manner is a change from the strategy of showing models posing alone in appealing outfits, but one that positions the consumer as "powerful and smart and stylish and sexy."[14]

Fat bodies, which used to be disciplined by simply refusing to publicly represent their excesses, are now tamed by domesticating the threat they pose to current beauty and health standards. Being deliberately, happily fat disturbs mainstream notions of attractiveness (e.g., nobody would desire to be fat, nobody would desire someone who is fat), so female fatness has been recuperated in the Mr. Big ads as a potential object of male affection.[15] Thus domesticated, "fit . . . into the dominant constructions of feminine appearances and roles," fat is made safe and unthreatening.[16] Case in point: Plus USA Woman pageant founder DeLores Pressley explains that the "pageant is much more than a pageant. . . . It's sort of like a coming out. . . . We're not advocates of obesity; we still want people to be healthy. But we also want to say, 'No matter how much you weigh, you can still look stunning with the right wardrobe, the right accessories.' "[17]

In some strange maneuver, the objectification against which feminists have been fighting for decades becomes the new dream state of the fat woman consumer. Charlotte Cooper discusses the availability of clothes and products for fat people as a consumer revolution[18]—but should fat people be so quick to measure success by being made into a commercial market? Isn't that what they're mad at the diet industry for doing to them? When faced with the seemingly paltry resources of abjection, the "elevated" state of being worshiped on a pedestal is something fat women frequently yearn for. But why is feminine fashion, deemed so frivolous by patriarchal society and by "serious" second-wave feminists alike, supposed to be the signal that fat women have arrived?

Fashion designers have claimed that "all women have three 'fashion rights': the right to look good, the right to wear attractive styles, and the right to be creative in fashion."[19] The language of rights used here detracts from more important rights, especially because these rights are couched within the impulses of capitalism. Yes, fat women have the right to spend just as much money as anyone else to look trendy. But how does this change their lives?

Fat feminist activists, contrary to expectations, often deny the notion that fashion is a tool of the patriarchy. Nomy Lamm, a fat, disabled, anarchist-feminist zine maker, believes that having fun with fashion is not the same as working toward society's beauty ideals; fashion, according to Lamm, can be used as a means of resistance and self-definition, a way of making a scene. "Why would I want to conform to some boring standard developed by capitalists and their lackeys when there are much more com-

pelling options? . . . The fashion industry tells me that I should wear flow-
ing drapery that hides my body, so my decision to wear miniskirts and
low-cut lingerie is a defiant and resounding 'Fuck you!' "[20] But what does
one make of Lamm's version of resistance when Lane Bryant, bastion of
capitalism that it is, showcases bare-midriff halter tops, sexy satin lingerie,
hip-hugging python-print pants, and over-the-top bustiers for fat women?
Capitalist enterprise seems to have consumed her revolution and is selling
it back to the public at a 200 percent retail markup.[21] However, Lamm's
insistence on having choices and the freedom to play with fashion does
illuminate the political nature of fashion.

In a stinging indictment of the difficulty of finding cool clothes for fat
bodies, Mariko Tamaki proclaims, "All well-dressed fat people should be
fucking worshipped and hailed as the Gods they are. Should I not choose
to walk around for the rest of my days angry and nude, I'm going to opt
instead to wear a t-shirt that says—'I'm a well-dressed fat person and I
deserve your respect for my efforts.' "[22] Her critique culminates in a blue-
print for her fashion revolution:

> I'll take my naked body to the streets in protest. I'll pummel the public with
> what it insists on denying and avoiding: tons of mountainous, sexy flesh. I'll
> bare my bare boobs and squish my sweaty bum at strangers. I'll squeak
> against every surface available and leave strange marks to embarrass the
> public. I'll gather an army of fat angry naked soldiers and we'll take to the
> streets. We'll go to the Gap and touch all their clothes and use up all their
> perfume samples till they agree to stock size 16 to 30 as standard practice.
> Look out . . . the revolution is coming.[23]

In response to such demands, couture fashionistas (as differentiated from
mall-based retailers like Lane Bryant) have begun to move away from the
brittle frames so popular on runway models in recent years. Paco Flaque,
director of the Salon Gaudi, Spain's annual fashion show, no longer wel-
comes models smaller than a British size 10, suggesting, "If we promote
the image of skinny women we are hurting our young people, and I am
against that."[24] Fat activist Marilyn Wann opposes the ban, arguing that
"instead of merely protecting our fragile egos from models with 30-inch
hips, he should let these waifs continue their work . . . but also include in
his show some models with 40-inch . . . or even 50-inch hips." She points
out that the subsequent outcry by the Spanish health ministry about the
unfairness of "illegalizing" thin people is hypocritical. "I can't recall the
last time a government official protested the lack of fat models in fashion

shows, much less the very real discrimination fat people face. . . . Isn't it equally unfair to 'illegalize,' or otherwise render invisible we-the-fat?"[25] Wann's observations reveal the extent to which fat women have failed to fully materialize as models on the runway or in other commercial contexts.

But even in the higher end of the fashion world, notorious for its attitude that "we don't worry about women who don't worry about themselves," plus-sized garments are becoming increasingly available. Why not throw on an Anne Klein leather coat ($1,050) with an Oscar de la Renta sequined T-shirt ($165), if you've managed to save up despite the pay penalty you endure for being fat?[26] Ophira Edut is suspicious, though, of this new accommodation: "Will equal access to haute couture lead to equal rights in the workplace, in health care and everywhere else size discrimination runs rampant?"[27]

Capitalist tensions abound in commercial attitudes toward fatness. Made-in-America ideological impulses drive women to be dissatisfied with their bodies, so they are encouraged to consume material mass-produced antidotes in the name of self-improvement. Thus, even fashion magazines that feature fat women "may continue to create and prey on women's anxieties in order to sell products, even while they purportedly relieve anxieties about being fat."[28] With the influx of fat-accepting commodities, fat folk are embraced as consuming subjects but not as social subjects.[29] David Ehrenstein, referring to gay consumers, says that "the market is there for the picking, and questions of 'morality' yield ever so briefly to the quest for capital."[30] In a similar vein, while it is still morally and aesthetically questionable in mainstream culture to deign fatness appealing in any way, the market is ripe—there are many women literally dying to feel their bodies are acceptable—and so any doubts are assuaged by the promise of monetary gain.

Erin Keating discusses the capitalist tensions at work in the world of plus-size fashion magazines. She argues that *Mode* is "a long-awaited counterbalance to the tried-and-true fashion formula that sells women dissatisfaction with their bodies and the goods and services that will abate that dissatisfaction. . . . *Mode* is proving that self-love can sell ad space and magazines as effectively as self-hatred."[31] However, Keating undermines her declaration by also pointing out the very limited notion of beauty marketed by the magazine; self-love then seems acceptable only if your self fits within the designated parameters, which for *Mode* is sizes

12–14–16. Her analysis of *Mode* recognizes that even though the editorial content features larger women than one would normally see in a fashion mag, the advertising content still features the same old skinny gals.

Referring to intentionally ambiguous advertising designed to appeal to straight and gay consumers alike, Danae Clark writes that "the sexual indeterminacy of gay window advertising's dual market approach . . . allows a space for lesbian identification, but must necessarily deny the representation of lesbian identity politics."[32] Advertising featuring persons with whom fat readers can identify is rarely indeterminate, given the visual nature of fatness. There doesn't seem to be the same obstacle present to representing fat identity politics as exists for lesbian identity politics. Perhaps that explains why media industries have been so reluctant for so long to put fat on display in any way that connotes acceptance; its presence too easily founds a fat-positive politics, the ramifications of which might be a negative impact on the health and beauty industries that fund them. One might examine a range of media strategies adopted in order to present fat in an anti-political way. Consider, for example, the fact that "plus-size" now refers to sizes 12, 14, and 16—the sizes worn by average-weight American women.[33] These average women surely aren't presented as political, just prettier than anyone had realized. Conveniently, their more sizable sisters are once again rendered invisible.

Nonetheless, it is possible to argue that fat itself (within a small range of size variation) has been made fashionable. The *Los Angeles Times* proclaims that "for a growing group that includes the ever-widening, fashion-conscious baby boomers, being large has become a statement of individuality and confidence."[34] We know this how? Because fat women can now buy clothes at a considerable markup for their size that make them look like everyone else. Oh, the irony!

It's even more ironic when one considers that, excepting celebrity spokespersons like Manheim and Latifah, models in fat-oriented magazines like *Mode* actually began *shrinking* in the 1990s.[35] Readers express consternation that size 8 models with large breasts are considered "plus" size, but retail apparel analysts respond that "no matter how much plus-size consumers complain about the stereotypes thrust upon them by mainstream retailers, they still don't want to look at the truly large-size models, in size 18 and up."[36] We seem to come to an impasse here in thinking about representation. The fashion industry won't feature fat models because the public apparently won't accept them, but the public stands little chance of being able to accept fat models until the fashion industry portrays them in the same flattering light they shine on their slimmer sisters. Edut echoes this sentiment, suggesting, "Maybe fashion is the tip of a much larger iceberg. Plus-size fashion might be a Band-Aid; it might be guerilla activism. After all, how can women stop cringing at our own curves and rolls unless we see them presented as 'normal' in the media?"[37]

Erin Keating argues that "visibility leads to acceptance in our seeing-is-believing culture." In trying to decide just how much praise to lavish on plus-size fashion mag *Mode*, Keating concludes that "market forces are driving what is essentially a political gain for women. If the personal is political, then being able to find clothes that fit and make you feel good about yourself is a political plus. In my mind, we must take these successes whether they come through direct action like marches and rallies, or through market recognition of yet another way to make a buck."[38]

Given the increasing superfluousness of people as producers, it is ever more important that we function competently as consumers. Thomas Szasz has pointed out how people have become the projects on which others can work. Obesity is a much-needed aesthetic and medical problem, in that it gives plenty of non-fat people something to work on.[39] What some of the more assimilationist early fat-acceptance leaders sought, then, was not a violent political revolt, but instead a peaceful consumer revolution—a happening that results in change based on the wishes of the consumer.

I want to be as hopeful as Keating and the assimilationist activists, but Danae Clark's assertion rings in my ears: "Style as resistance becomes commodifiable as chic when it leaves the political realm and enters the fashion world. This simultaneously diffuses the political edge of style. Resistant trends . . . become restyled as high-priced fashion."[40] Indeed, fat women demanding the right to wear stylish clothes seems like a compromised victory, unless one considers how they have developed strategies of choice and subversion to bring consumer culture more in line with their *own* desires, rather than the ones instilled in them by commerce. Fat women *do* assert themselves, making visible their subjectivities, in inventive ways not expected by the peddlers of plus-sized togs.

Consumer society has generated processes that make it harder for any specific group to impose its preferred hierarchy of valuable bodies across society. "The rapid internalization and circulation of consumer and 'lifestyle' goods threatens the readability of those signs used by the dominant to signify their elite physical capital."[41] When fat people are no longer relegated to unflattering tent-dresses made of inferior fabrics, when they look more like their slim counterparts in terms of appealing garb, there's one less thing to dismiss them for. But when they disdain "blending in" in favor of cobbling together a look from the scattered resources available and becoming more brave about appearing in ways that defy the "tasteful" intentions of the commodifiers of corpulence, fashion *is* revolutionary; its newfound ability stymies fat oppression.

6

. . . .

Framing Fatness: Popular Representations of Obesity as Disability

What do obesity and more familiar subsets of disability have in common? According to disability scholar Rosemarie Garland-Thomson, "disability . . . is the attribution of corporeal deviance—not so much a property of bodies as a product of cultural rules about what bodies should be or do."[1] Fat people, in their excessive refusal to be disciplined into culturally "acceptable" body shapes and sizes, are then as corporeally deviant as those others considered, without a second thought, to be disabled. For some, the difference lies in the perceived ability to control the conditions of one's disability. Many fat activists have resisted political affiliation with disability activists, despite significant commonalities, because of the double whammy of stigma that such a liaison might incur. Michael Bérubé thus accurately suggests, in his introduction to the work of Simi Linton, that "claiming disability is sure to become one of the most politically sensitive endeavors a body can undertake."[2]

Obesity is one of the most interesting inclusions in the Rehabilitation

Act of 1973 and the Americans with Disabilities Act of 1990. Though fat Americans are legally protected against discrimination so long as their condition substantially limits at least one of their major life activities or is perceived as doing so, controversy abounds about whether the condition of obesity, over which individuals are usually thought to have some personal control, should be protected. In this chapter, I explore the ways in which popular representations of fatness are implicated in battles both to claim and to exclude obesity as a disabling condition. I analyze these representations in an attempt to explicate their social and political significance to both disability politics and to a culture deeply invested in marginalizing difference.

History is long on representations of fat people, though their depiction is typically quite limited in scope. Popular images of fat men include the wealthy, politically powerful "fat cat," the sweetly avuncular Santa Claus type, and the funny guy, à la John Belushi, Chris Farley, and Louie Anderson. In few representations is fatness framed as a disability; certainly, it functions as a source of hilarity for some and a reassuring reminder of domestic life for others, but one must look to more recent representations to find connections between disability and fatness. Draw your own connections from Susan Peters's description of the representation of people with disabilities:

> From Victorian times, Western fiction and drama have portrayed tarnished images of people with disabilities which mirror and magnify prevalent societal perceptions. Predominant among these tarnished images are characteristics of disabled people as helpless, useless, pitiable, undesirable. They are dependent, incomplete in body and basic experiences of personhood. Disabled women are submissive, asexual, bitter and full of self-loathing. In short, disabled men and women are victims of societal misperceptions and of their own inability to reject and transcend the prejudice of others.[3]

Feature films of the 1990s, including *Heavy* (directed by James Mangold) and *Sweetie* (directed by Jane Campion), begin to sketch characters whose fatness (among other differences) creates a social disability for them. The main character in *Heavy*, a painfully shy fat man who lives with his mother, is threatened by social interaction, in part because he anticipates that his body will garner only rejection. In *Sweetie*, our heroine is fat and unabashedly sexual, quite unlike the fellow in *Heavy*; Sweetie's aggressive sexuality does not seem to fit appropriately with her fat body— it is as if she fails to realize that her body is not culturally acceptable for

sexual appreciation—and as a result of her "misfit" status, she is understood to be mentally ill. Sweetie's framework for understanding the relation between her body and her actions is skewed, says society.

Other popular media forms of the late twentieth century reinforce the
idea of fatness as socially disabling. One interesting forum for such propaganda is the daytime talk or variety show, including *The Rosie
O'Donnell Show*, *Oprah*, and *The Roseanne Show*. Pay attention not to
the guests or the topics discussed but to the weight loss travails of any of
the hosts, and you will recognize a pervasive discourse in which fatness
is denigrated. Though O'Donnell, Winfrey, and Barr utilize mantras of
weight loss in pursuit of good health, all refer to the sense of shame
engendered by a failure to live up to social expectations about their appearance, particularly given their prominence in the "looks-happy" entertainment industry.

Beyond talk shows lie prime-time bastions of fat imagery such as *The
Practice* and *The Drew Carey Show*, each of which present both a fat
male and a fat female character. With the exception of Mimi on *Drew
Carey*, whose frightful, caricatured appearance and brash interpersonal
manner also arguably provoke social disability, fatness plays an insignificant role in the existence of the other three characters (Drew, Jimmy
Berluti, or Ellenor Frutt). These are competent, funny, interesting characters who, amazingly, have sexual relationships with (non-fat) others,
say intelligent things, and generally lead full lives; they also just happen
to be fat. Many fat activists cite these characters as marking progress in
the creation of a repertoire of "positive" media images for fat viewers to
draw on when developing their own self-concept, unlike other, unidi-
mensional, depictions where fat is the most telling thing about a given
character.

Rosemarie Garland-Thomson's concept of the "normate" is useful for
understanding the stakes in propping up one-dimensional representations
of fat people. The normate represents those figures who command power
based on a combination of bodily configurations and cultural capital;
their power is maintained through the deployment of standards of beauty,
fitness, and normalcy which celebrate some bodies at the expense of others. Garland-Thomson concludes that

> the meanings attributed to extraordinary bodies reside not in inherent phys-
> ical flaws, but in social relationships in which one group is legitimated by
> possessing valued physical characteristics and maintains its ascendancy and

its self-identity by systematically imposing the role of cultural or corporeal inferiority on others. Representation thus simultaneously buttresses an embodied version of normative identity and shapes a narrative of corporeal difference that excludes those whose bodies or behaviors don't conform.[4]

My intention, then, is to examine closely two relatively complex representations of fatness as both physical and social disability, in order to consider how such treatments add to or subtract from an abnormalizing discourse. First, I will discuss an episode of *The Simpsons* in which Homer gains sixty-one pounds in an attempt to classify as disabled; then I will move to an examination of the feature film *What's Eating Gilbert Grape?* and its representation of a reclusive but loving fat woman.

A useful framework for such an endeavor is provided in the work of Paul Darke on cinematic representations of disability. Darke draws on the statistical analysis work of Cumberbatch and Negrine, whose analysis of disability images he claims is significant "in identifying the prevalence with which disability is represented either in a medical context or as something which one 'bravely' overcomes in a struggle to be 'normal.' "[5] Darke eschews the vocabulary of "positive" or "negative" representations, claiming that *positive* usually equates with more "normalized" images, which ultimately "validate not difference but normality, the very illusion at the heart of the oppression of disabled people."[6] He further suggests that "abnormality is used in cultural imagery to define the parameters of normality," and investigates the genre of representations that deploys disabled characters to confront imagined threats to the hegemony of normalcy. Darke concludes that "for a largely 'normal' audience viewing a normality drama, an able-bodied audience's cultural and social baggage will be almost exclusively rooted in the socially hegemonic interpretation of impairment as a medical and individual 'problem' to be either overcome or eradicated."[7]

Consider, then, this episode of *The Simpsons*: during morning calisthenics at his unsavory job at the nuclear power plant, notoriously lazy Homer Simpson hears of a coworker whose on-the-job accident earned him full pay for no work during his recovery. Homer, green with envy, proceeds to tempt the fates toward his own accident, to no avail. He fails to harm himself in any significant way. Next, we see Homer pondering a pamphlet called *Am I Disabled?* Realizing the elusiveness of conditions like "Juggler's Remorse," he happily sets his sights on "Hyperobesity," for which the minimum weight is three hundred pounds.

When his socially conscious and unusually responsible daughter Lisa hears of his plan, she cries, "You're abusing a program intended to help the unfortunate. . . . Obesity is really unhealthy, any doctor will tell you that." With his regular doctor seconding Lisa's opinion, Homer visits Dr. Nick, the quack graduate of Hollywood Upstairs Medical College. Nick recommends a slow, steady gorging process, aided by a focus on "the neglected food groups—the whipped, the congealed, and the chocotastic." He enlightens Homer about the food-rubbing test, wherein a transparent grease stain caused by rubbing his food on test paper is his "window to weight gain."

In the next shots, we see Homer pigging out, even buying vitamin store weight-gain supplements, and weighing himself regularly. A dream sequence interrupts, wherein a very rotund Homer works from his backyard, waltzes his wife Marge across the yard, and relishes his life, in contrast to his neighbor, the harried, work-a-day Flanders. After the dream sequence, we witness Homer's shopping spree at "The Vast Waistband," where his purchase of a flowered muumuu ensures his departure from the 9- to 5- work world.

When Marge, typically caring and patient, discovers Homer's scheme, she asks if Homer has thought about his health or his appearance. Later, she tells him he's setting a bad example for the kids, and she's finding him less physically attractive. Meanwhile, mischievous son Bart dreams of becoming "a lardo on workers' compensation just like Dad." Homer responds by defending himself and his new lifestyle choice, exclaiming that he's no longer lazy; he's now "a big fat dynamo!" Soon afterward, neighborhood children are peering in the window at Homer on the sofa, mocking his girth. Lisa defends Homer, now so immobile that he cannot close the shade.

Thus begins Homer's odyssey into fat oppression: he attempts to attend a movie but is denied access on the grounds that he will not fit in the seats. Onlookers make fun of him. Homer stands up for himself, suggesting that fat people are as smart and hardworking as anyone else, but then ironically returns home to discover that the pecking-bird toy he had left in charge of his job has let him down: his monitor suggests imminent danger at the plant. Fearing an explosion, Homer attempts to call the plant, but his fingers are too fat to dial. When he tries to jump in the car to head to the plant, his weight bursts the tires. Finally able to commandeer a passing ice cream truck, Homer makes it to the plant on time to plug the explosion with his fat body. The evil plant owner, Mr. Burns, gratefully asks Homer how he can repay him, and Homer pleads, "Make me thin again." Burns acts as physical trainer to Homer, but when Homer proves incapable of even a single sit-up, Burns snarls, "I'll just pay for the blessed liposuction." Homer shouts "Yahoo!" and the credits roll.

While *The Simpsons* is clearly a comedy, and a satirically subversive one at that, interesting, politically significant representations of fatness also exist in more serious texts, such as the 1993 film *What's Eating Gilbert Grape?* Reviewer Chris Hicks writes that Gilbert Grape (played by Johnny Depp) "is the most 'normal' character in the movie."[8] He's surrounded by eccentrics, including his developmentally disabled younger brother (Arnie, played by Leonardo DiCaprio) and his five-hundred-pound-plus mother (Momma, played by Darlene Cates) who has not left the house in seven years. Gilbert is the dutiful son and brother who forges a "career" at the local mom-and-pop grocer, which faces competition from the sparkling new chain store in the area. The disabilities of Momma and Arnie play off of each other in an interesting manner. When we first see Momma, she is being served a huge breakfast by one of her daughters; in most of the film's early scenes, Momma is shown eating, but she is always in her house. Arnie, on the other hand, likes to make a spectacle of himself. He frequently climbs the rural town's water tower, which draws not only the police and the Grape family, to get him down, but a crowd of curious onlookers as well. Arnie's disability is as spectacular and visible as Momma's is hidden away.

Gilbert's relationship to both Momma and Arnie is noteworthy. While he regularly engages in acts of caretaking for both of them, his comments to others reveal his frustration with the limitations of this role. In a voice-over about Arnie, Gilbert tells us, "Sometimes you want him to live, sometimes you don't." Gilbert also helps some neighbor kids by lifting them to the window to peer in at Momma's massive body. When a friend inquires about Momma, Gilbert replies that "she's fat," as if that is all one needs to know. Gilbert carries out his duties but quietly seethes with a sort of resigned resentment. The disabled people in his life fail to provide him with much pleasure. Instead, it is rail-thin women who distract Gilbert from his woes, in the form of married-but-cheating housewife Betty Carver (played by Mary Steenburgen) and enigmatic Airstream traveler Becky (played by Juliette Lewis).

One of the key subplots of the film involves the Grape family's preparations for Arnie's eighteenth birthday party, a special event because Arnie was not predicted to survive this long. In one scene, Momma discusses recipes for the party with her daughters, and Arnie goes out of control, laughing and shouting "Dad is dead!" Momma, unable to bear it any longer, stops Arnie by stomping on the floor, and Gilbert notices the floorboards giving way beneath her. In a later scene, Momma returns from the bathroom to her favorite spot on the couch, and the sound effects that accompany her steps across the floor are of gargantuan proportions. When Momma falls asleep in front of the television, as she usually does, her children try to convince her to sleep in her bed, ostensibly for her own comfort but really out of concern that the floor is going to cave in from the continuous pressure of her weight.

In a related subplot, Gilbert and his sweetheart, Becky, discuss the idea of beauty. Becky, embarrassed by her grandmother's insistence that Becky is a beautiful young woman, tells Gilbert that physical beauty is highly overrated. She believes that "it's what you *do* that matters," instead of what you look like. She asks Gilbert about what he wants to do in life, whether he wants to move away. Gilbert replies, "We'd like to move but my mom is pretty much attached to the house; she's wedged in." He then tells Becky that Momma is like a beached whale. Later on, Gilbert refuses to allow Becky to visit the house and meet Momma; it seems that Arnie's disability, with which Becky is already familiar, is enough, and that Becky encountering Momma might be too much to bear.

Meanwhile, back at the house, we are treated to several shots of Momma "mothering" Arnie—calling him cute names, cuddling with him, and fretting over his whereabouts when he's not in the immediate vicinity. As the story progresses, we realize that Momma's concern is not baseless, for Arnie has once again endangered himself by running off to climb the water tower. This time, though, the police take Arnie into custody, citing the failure of his family to keep him out of trouble. It is exactly the spectacle of Arnie's disability as manifest in his final climb of the tower that forces Momma's body to morph from specter to spectacle as well. Upon hearing of Arnie's detainment by the police, Momma realizes that only she can free him. She decides to leave the house after a seven-year incumbency. Yelling "Get my coat!" Momma heads for the family car. Down at the station, she storms down the hall, startling all who cross her path, shouting for the police captain. When she finds him, Momma tells him that she has come for her son, utterly defiant in the face of proper procedures. She demands, "Give me my son." Surprisingly, Arnie is relinquished to her. When the family steps out of the station into the light of day, we see that a crowd has gathered to watch Momma's public appearance. Onlookers laugh, jeer, and gape. A camera clicks: evidence of her deviance is captured on film. When Momma returns home, she appears listless and no longer appears to have any appetite.

Soon, Arnie's party gets under way. While his sisters work on the cake and the decorations, Momma voices her reluctance to be seen at the party; she declares that she will remain inside and watch from the window. Indeed, she does remain in her bedroom during the festivities. Gilbert returns home after an episode in which he hits and then abandons Arnie, and seeks forgiveness from his mother. Momma, angry with Gilbert, reminds him that Arnie is just "a helpless boy." She then tells Gilbert that she knows what a burden she is and that she is aware that he is ashamed of her. "I never meant to be like this. I never wanted to be a joke." When Gilbert, who has had a change of heart after his run-in with Arnie, says that he wants Momma to meet Becky, Momma demurs; she's afraid of being hurt. Nonetheless, Gilbert brings Becky into the room. Momma quickly announces, "I haven't always been like this," and Becky endearingly responds in kind: "Well, I haven't always been like *this*."

After the party, perhaps invigorated by her meeting with Becky, Momma decides to ascend the stairs, much to the surprise of her family. After an arduous struggle up the steps, Momma makes her way to a bedroom, where she dies on the bed. When the family realizes, they call the police; they are repelled when a radio dispatcher says that it will require either the National Guard or a crane to extricate her body from the house. Gilbert's sister cries, fearing the appearance of a crowd for such an event. Gilbert exclaims, "I'm not going to let her be a joke," a statement that has extra resonance because of his earlier conversation with the town mortician's son, who reveals that the undertakers make fun of the corpses of unattractive people. The family moves all of the furniture out to the lawn as Gilbert douses their home in gasoline and strikes a match. Momma is immolated. The film ends with Gilbert, who had previously felt trapped in the house and the role of caretaker, smiling and promising Arnie that they are free to go anywhere they want now.

In beginning to unpack these dense characterizations, one must ask a number of questions. How do Momma and fat Homer stack up against those disabled with "the temerity to emerge as forthright and resourceful people, nothing like the self-loathing, docile, bitter or insentient fictional versions" to which the public has grown accustomed?[9] Is Momma despondent about her situation or indignant at the way society treats her? What about Homer? What models of disability are most closely associated with these characters: pariah, social and economic liability, tolerant utilization, or something more promising?[10] In these popular texts, which characters are "depicted as draining pleasure from others or are themselves compromised in their ability to experience pleasure"?[11] How does the abnormality of these characters reify the parameters of the normal?

First, consider the self-concepts of Momma and Homer. Homer is entirely happy being fat, and a number of times he champions the notion that fat people can be just as vital as anyone else. Of course, in the end, he reverts to his usual "svelte" 239 pounds, probably as a result of Marge's sexual disdain and the realization that working from home was not all it was cracked up to be. Momma, on the other hand, has deeply internalized society's revulsion for fat bodies; she sadly laments her enormity and her burden on Gilbert. Her moment of bravery comes in her public promenade at the police station, as she defies the mandate that the unsightliness of fat be hidden out of view. Still, by the end of the film, moments before her death, all she can muster is an apology for her own existence. While both contain inspired moments that challenge fat oppression, both ultimately capitulate to agendas that reinforce the disabling of bodies marked by difference.

Indeed, both characters are represented in the fashion of some of the more discouraging models of disability introduced by J. R. Hanks and L. M. Hanks Jr. in 1948 and reworked by Simi Linton.[12] Momma exists as a pariah to most of the community, in that she is rarely seen and seems to be trapped in her own home. She is a social and economic liability for the family, in particular for Gilbert, who must work at Larson's store to support her and who is embarrassed to have his girlfriend meet her. The best we can say about Momma is perhaps that there is tolerant utilization of her by the neighbor boys, who watch her through the window for entertainment purposes, though of course Momma gets nothing in return. In *The Simpsons*, Homer is not quite a pariah, though a newspaper headline after his disability "send-off" reads, "Burns survives brush with shut-in," a sardonic comment on the ease with which his type is read as an outcast. Homer is somewhat of an economic liability for his company, in that they have to set him up to work at home and continue to pay him, despite their inability to monitor his work. (Regular watchers of *The Simpsons*, however, realize that Homer's economic liability to his employer has little to do with his new disability, and more to do with his long-term incompetence.) At best, Homer is granted limited participation in his culture; he can work, but he is physically segregated, and because of his inability to adapt or fit, he is limited in his choice of recreational pursuits.

Both Homer and Momma are depicted as powerful pleasure drains on those surrounding them. The only character to whom Momma seems capable of providing pleasure is Arnie, a developmentally disabled character who is represented as delighted by anyone who is nice to him. Though there are hints that Becky enjoys her company, their scene together is so underdeveloped that we never really get a strong sense of this. Gilbert certainly seems to suffer because of Momma's existence; it is only after her death that he smiles easily and speaks happily of his newfound freedom. Homer, in becoming fat, is depicted as depriving Marge of sexual pleasure. However, he does provide a kind of pleasure to Bart, who idolizes him as a role model for deviance par excellence. Though there are some pleasures to be taken from these fat characters, they are obviously compromised pleasures.

Finally, I want to examine how the abnormality of fat Homer and Momma serve to reinforce normality as superior. Recall the movie reviewer's contention that Gilbert is "the most 'normal' character in the movie." Without the freaky sideshow of "retarded" Arnie and "morbidly obese" Momma, what would a viewer make of Gilbert, with his apparent lack of ambition, stalled affair with a married woman, simple-minded friends, and small-town ignorance about the world? Gilbert himself is no box of chocolates; he only appears so because of his positioning between his abnormal mother and brother. Interestingly, the movie ends a year after Momma's death, with Gilbert still sticking around in his town of Endora; he *dreams* of moving on but in fact is so complacent that he has remained in his dead-end world. The movie *has* to end there; otherwise, how would we understand Gilbert-as-stuck without Momma as his anchor?

Homer's temporary fatness, it seems, weighs on his character in a different manner. While Homer is typically inept and lazy in other episodes, his fatness-as-disability has the unexpected effect of making him a happier, better worker. Because the show is a comedy, the culturally unappealing device of weight gain is stood on its head; Homer is noble only in his obesity. The generic conventions of the sitcom require that our expectations about good and bad, superior and inferior, be temporarily subverted. We laugh, safely confident that Homer really is a knucklehead and that the reasonable voices of Marge and Lisa ultimately prevail: fatness is irresponsible, unhealthy, and undesirable.

I hope to have examined these texts in sufficient detail to be able to estimate their usefulness to a revolution of disabled bodies. I believe that neither *The Simpsons* nor *What's Eating Gilbert Grape?* are purely "negative" depictions of obesity as disability; both contain interesting complexities notable in a growing canon of disability representations. Ultimately, though, I am afraid that both texts do the cultural work of further socially disabling fat bodies.

I agree with Bickenbach, who is cited in the work of British disability activists Jane Campbell and Mike Oliver: "Counter-hegemonic politics is far more revolutionary than political agitation directed at specific legislative or political ends. The aim of the former is to attack, directly and dramatically, a dominant societal framework, rather than to use it and the social institutions that make it up in order to win favourable concessions."[13] I believe that analyzing the grammar of images that conspire to disenfranchise some human bodies is vital and important political work. Scholarly efforts at reframing popular representations contribute much to dismantling the barriers to the social integration of all sorts of "revolting" bodies.

7

. . . .

The Queerness of Fat

Queens will not be pawns.
DEREK JARMAN

The media brouhaha of the late twentieth century over the search for a fat gene mirrors the parallel and contemporaneous controversy about the causes of homosexuality. We've heard about genes, hormones, fear of being sexually attractive, and dozens of other causes for fatness and homosexuality, each one advanced with the understanding that finding a remedy would be a financially rewarding proposition. Why, though, do we need to explain (away) these modes of being, when few scientists are hard at work on finding the cause for slenderness or heterosexuality? When we engage in cause-seeking rhetoric, we presume that some intervention into the "problem" is necessary.[1] Still, questions continue to rear their heads in regard to both body size and sexual proclivity as trendy theories come and go. Are they lifestyle preferences over which individuals have considerable control? Or are they hardwired into our biology, offering us little choice in the matter? In the "lifestyle preference" camp, fatness is thought to be the result of a defense mechanism—

that individual weight gain is usually a symptom of other underlying problems.

Michelle Levine's *I Wish I Were Thin, I Wish I Were Fat,* for example, attempts to persuade readers that diets fail because of powerful but unconscious fears of thinness that stem from a belief that fatness is safe while thinness is beautiful, and thus hated, making slender people a rather lonely lot.[2] Robert Pool, in *FAT: Fighting the Obesity Epidemic,* views obesity as "a disease caused by a sick environment to which some of us are more susceptible than others."[3] Though the disease is supposedly caused by something outside our control, he believes that the remedy is certainly within our powers, arguing that readers should build their willpower and seek help from the latest diet fads when useful.

The idea that fatness is a form of physical protection against sexual demands is also influential in both popular and scholarly literature. From Susie Orbach's paperbacks to the academic journals of many social-scientific disciplines, we read that "some women who are survivors of sexual abuse . . . hope that by being 'big' and by not fitting into the cultural ideal of beautiful, no sexual attraction and consequently no sexual assault can occur."[4] A recent article in *Moxie* magazine told the story of a young woman who gained a significant amount of weight after being raped. She explains the utility of fatness in a troubling, and incorrect, passage: "Fat girls don't get raped. Fat girls aren't attractive. Fat girls are invisible because fat girls aren't attractive. My fat protects and redeems me, but I've come to realize that my fat also victimizes me."[5] Well, sadly, fat women *do* get raped, and rape has nothing to do with attraction. But the most unfortunate misconception on the part of this most unfortunate woman is that it is her fat that is victimizing her. Instead, I submit that it is her attitude that dooms her; she stands to learn from the way queers have countered similar claims about the source of their difficulties.

While both queers and fat folk are understood as manifesting symptoms to mask a more difficult underlying problem, they also share a reputation for sexual deviance. Work on social stigma reports that stigmatized individuals are typically depicted as a composite of three overwhelming characteristics: animalistic, hypersexual, and overvisible.[6] Gay men are suspected of sexually predatory behavior and maligned for "flaunting" their desires in front of a straight audience that would, it seems, prefer temporary blindness. Similarly, it takes little imagination to conjure up "pig" or "cow" as a popular term of insult for fat people, and their reputed sexual desperation is the stuff of legend (not to mention numerous 1980s teen-sex romp flicks). The in-your-face visibility of fat bodies seals the deal. The homosexual is stigmatized, obviously, in the arena of sexuality, though surprisingly that is where a great deal of fat stigma also manifests itself.

Even amidst efforts to ameliorate the Puritan legacy of sexual hangups, fat people suffer unnerving stigmatization. While the 1972 release of *The Joy of Sex* was a step forward to opening people's eyes to a variety of sexual practices, the decision of author Alex Comfort to list fat in the "Problems" section was not helpful to the budding fat acceptance movement. More offensive than Comfort's racist tale of pretty fat girls who must "resort" to Middle Eastern boyfriends is his narrow-minded mandate: "If you are grossly overweight, set about losing it, whether you value your sex life or only your life."[7]

A generous reader might understand that this command seems to emanate from his assumption that obesity causes impotence in men. However, a more critical reader would question the need to lose weight—especially for fat women, whom Comfort claims are better suited to rear-entry sex and sex on a hard surface than are thinner women. If there are absolutely no sexual drawbacks—only advantages—for fat women listed in *The Joy of Sex*, why then would weight loss improve their sex lives? The stigma, unwarranted by Comfort's other claims, is a holdover from a culture that continues to revile fat women's bodies for ostensibly aesthetic (but entirely political) reasons.

Psychologist Nita McKinley contends that society imposes strict limits on women's desires: "The only 'indulgence' allowed us is a low-calorie product. Thus, a woman who is fat is doubly sexually deviant: she must be engaging in sex (eating) for her own pleasure and she presumably displays a voracious appetite. A woman with ideal weight, on the other hand, has more appropriate[ly] controlled her appetites."[8] The double meaning for plumpness in women traces to the turn of the twentieth century, when the extra fatness of criminal women, such as prostitutes, was thought to signify their "natural tendency to their craft."[9]

Catherine Manton confirms this double whammy for women in her discussion of 1950s psychoanalytic theory, which aligned appetite for food with repressed appetite for sex. In order to avoid the stigma, women were turned off of both sex and food, lest they be accused of insatiable, and culturally unacceptable, lust.[10] The conflation of appetites for food with appetites for sex is not a dusty historical relic, however; interpretations of more modern popular culture texts, like the 1980s TV show starring Pee-wee Herman, operate on the same premise. Queer theorist Alexander Doty postulates that because Pee-wee's 1950s sissy boy can't take direct erotic notice of butch male characters on the show, fat women are used as "beards" for Pee-wee's desires. The characters of Mrs. René and Mrs. Steve, both fat and food-obsessed, are understood as representing Pee-wee's sexual frustrations.[11] Though Doty is simply drawing on a familiar cultural repertoire to render his interpretation, it is nonetheless frustrating that fatness stands in for sexual frustration once again, even in an otherwise inventive and forward-thinking series.

In her classic study *Fat and Thin: A Natural History of Obesity*, Anne Scott Beller interrogates the cultural contention that fat women, because they are viewed as morally and sexually repulsive and are thought to be frigid as a result of that treatment, are unlikely to have active and satisfying sex lives. Beller declares that the assumption failed to test out and that in fact, fat women outscored thin women by two to one on "erotic readiness" and "general sexual excitability."[12] While it's not news to some people that fat is sexy, the publication of her report helped to lend credence to a widely disbelieved truth. Unfortunately, though, Beller throws the power to judge sexiness back to the hangmen: "Are fat women sexier? Perhaps the last word on this subject will have to come from men; judgments about erotic desirability are, like most other matters of taste, largely in the eye of the beholder."[13] That *women* cannot evaluate other women's sex appeal is problematic, but this problem is trumped by the fact that power has been taken from women to determine *their own* sexiness.

There is a self-fulfilling prophecy at work in the denigration of fat people that can lead to disturbances in their interpersonal and sexual relationships. Because the social environment fails to support the idea of fat as personally and sexually appealing, the continuous insults to which they are subject may do psychic damage to fat people. Twenty years ago, an article in the *British Journal of Sexual Medicine* alleged that "the obese have unconsciously given up the struggle to preserve a non-derogatory attitude toward themselves,"[14] an act that makes fat oppression an even easier cultural accomplishment. I believe that fat activists must continue to take cues from queer activists about how to persist in this uphill battle.

Queer acceptance/activism and fat acceptance/activism have much in common, given that fatness may be read as a mere subset of queerness.

Because fat people are not supposed to be sexy or sexual, "any sex involving a fat person is by definition 'queer,' no matter what the genders of any of the partners involved."[15] Inasmuch as fat accentuates the size and shape of certain sexualized body parts, some folks find fat people more masculine or feminine than their thinner counterparts.[16]

There are advantages and disadvantages to fat activists aligning with other oppressed minority groups, such as members of racial and ethnic minority groups. The upside is protection of civil liberties, generation of support and legitimacy, and improved mobilization; the downside involves a sustained focus on the stigmatized identity, as well as politics of a somewhat assimilatory stripe.[17] But as the civil liberties of queers are *not* fully protected, and as their politics (as contrasted with gay or lesbian rights movements) are rarely assimilatory, a casual observer might have a difficult time gauging the benefits of queering fat politics.

After all, queer circles generally provide little refuge from the sizism that permeates mainstream culture, and in fact foster anti-fat bias to a greater extent, especially among men. Gay writer Patrick Giles laments: "Despite GMHC, ACT UP, 12-steps, Louise, Larry, and crystals, I don't find our community more sensitive since AIDS and activism. We are as deeply obsessed with appearance and 'normality' as we've ever been. Clonism has been succeeded by gym bodies, little-boy bodies and ACT UP *couture*. Ostracism of big men thrives."[18]

Popular belief reassures us that men are allowed to grow fat with much less anxiety than women, but according to Ganapati Durgadas, fat feminizes men in a potentially dangerous manner. The roundness and softness of fat men confirms their "womanishness"—meaning "you can be fucked, in more ways than one, within the patriarchal hierarchy as your relative male status is revoked."[19] Durgadas argues that while fatness feminizes heterosexual men, its feminizing effect on gay and bisexual men is more profound: "Fat gay and bisexual men . . . are less like men and more like women. Fleshy bulk or stoutness in females implies inappropriate strength or toughness. In males, it represents womanlike weakness or physical impressionability. We are reminders of the feminine stigma with which heterosexism still tars queer men."[20]

Despite Durgadas's implication that fat women might be more popular in lesbian scenes because of their perceived strength, one needs only to peruse the personal ads of the local progressive weekly to see this is not necessarily the truth.[21] But when fat *is* embraced in queer circles, it is taken up quite differently by lesbians and gay men. Researcher Alex Robertson Textor, in analyzing fat-positive magazines created within both communities, finds that gay men's media simplify and fetishize this sexual difference, while lesbian zines radically politicize it. "The dynamic, complicated debates featured in *Fat Girl* are not to be found within *Bulk Male* or *Big Ad*—largely, I believe, because gay male cultural politics have not been founded upon an engagement with as sweepingly radical an analysis as lesbian cultural politics have been."[22] Sexuality activist Joël Barraquiel Tan posits that this difference might also stem from the visual orientation and heightened body consciousness of gay men: "If fat is a feminist issue, then fat or heft is a fetishized one for gay men. Gay men have a tendency to sexualize difference, where lesbians have historically politicized it."[23]

Though there's plenty of disdain for fat in queer circles, I remain interested in the promise offered by queer communities for enhancing fat politics. Supportive queer communities nurture their members, whatever size or shape, recognizing that "to be cruel, dismissive, or judgmental of each other plays into the hands of those who actively promote an antigay agenda."[24] One queer subculture marked by fat acceptance is Girth and Mirth. Though not an intentionally political group—more of a social one, instead—the organization's embrace of a more generous aesthetic promises a rethinking of the fat body as sexy, which is ultimately a political move for a marginalized community.

Textor examines the dynamics of the big men's movement as articulated in the publications it has produced and argues that big men's media not only reflect a celebration of and desire for fat bodies, but are spaces where desires themselves are produced.[25] The primary formal social and organizational vehicle for this production of desires has been the Girth and Mirth Club, started in 1976, and its attendant media outlets, including websites like Chubnet, pornographic videos, and magazines like *Big Ad* and *Bulk Male*.[26] Textor suggests that the historical feminization of fat men has precipitated an allied effort to masculinize them within the gay male cultural context, and such efforts are borne out in their media representations.

Textor exposes the overlaps between big men and bears as gay male identity categories. Bears, frequently understood as large and hirsute, are thought to be aligned with big men in their "rebellion against the emphasis on physical perfection, which pervades that gay community."[27] What counts as a bear is defined through recourse to connotations: "a large or husky body, heavy body hair, a lumbering gait, an epicurean appetite, an attitude of imperturbability, a contented self-acceptance of his own masculinity."[28] In their alignment by rejection, big men and bears are inherently queer, as defined by rejection of mainstream standards, regardless of their sexual practices.

However, both bears and big men frequently reject each other. A big man suspicious of bear motives writes, "Somehow, naming yourself a 'bear' has come to mean that you don't have to face the fact [that] you're fat. It mitigates the stigma of being overweight and therefore obscures being 'out' as a gay CHUBBY, or, for those of you who don't like that term, FAT gay man."[29] Big men also often recognize bears as dependent upon the performance of a hypertraditional masculinity that many big men find regressive and marginalizing. Bears, for their part, often denigrate big men as insufficiently masculine and as having let themselves go. Witness the words of Ray Kampf, whose *Bear Handbook* chides, "There is a faction of heavyset men who will use the excuse 'I'm a Bear' to justify overeating. . . . Trying to bulk up is not the way to improve your Bear status. There is a line that is crossed when you realize you are no longer a Bear, but graduate to Girth and Mirth."[30] Les Wright, author of *The Bear Book*, sounds the alarm at what has happened in bear circles, where conformity, consumerism, and competition seem to have taken over a formerly inclusive space[31]—a move that threatens the politicization of fatness.

So how is the revaluation of fat gay male identity accomplished through media? Textor argues for *Bulk Male* that its "main purpose is to recharge fat gay men as sexually valuable. This recharge is delivered through the valuation of fat men as masculine."[32] In contrast, the more politicized *Big Ad* "eroticizes fat men while retaining mass itself as a primary and shared erotic denominator."[33]

Even in non-avowedly queer cultural spaces, body mass is eroticized, albeit in a less joyous, more secretive and guilty kind of way. The existence of fat admirers—usually average-weight men with a keen erotic interest in fat women—presents a remarkable dilemma for fat people interested in revaluing fatness. The unspeakable desires of fat admirers are widely regarded suspiciously by fat feminists as controlling, deviant, and fetishistic.[34] But what do fat folk stand to gain from an embrace of the attention lavished upon them by fat admirers? If fat feminists malign admirers just as the rest of society does, nothing is gained—fatness is seen as something one must be sick to admire. This may account for the number of fat admirers who closet their preference, feel uncomfortable about their desire, and thus treat the objects of their desire poorly.[35] If fat admiration could come out of the closet as just another part of sexuality—a lesson learned from the queers of Girth and Mirth—things might be better for fat women in the long run.

Fatness and queerness also share a concern for the politics of outing. In an interesting study of ritual conversation among girls of all ages, Mimi Nichter claims that the phrase "I'm so fat" serves as a beacon of reassurance that indeed one is *not* fat. The expression signifies personal and cultural concerns, and functions as an idiom of distress, a call for support from peers, a defense mechanism that allows its speaker to reveal her weak spots before others can do so, and a bonding device. Uttering "I'm so fat" solidifies group identity among girls whom a neutral observer would be hard-pressed to understand as fat. Unsurprisingly, girls who are truly fat don't engage in such fat talk, because to do so would "out" them.[36]

A politics of outing similar to that debated in queer communities exists in fat communities.[37] Public figures can be grouped into three categories based on their position vis-à-vis their own fatness: (1) Out and About; (2) Silent Types; (3) Traitors. Those who are Out and About publicly acknowledge their own fatness and typically embrace it. Actor Camryn Manheim, she of "This is for all the fat girls!" Emmy fame, would be a poster child for the group. Even poster children, though, have their share of internal contradictions. Despite the visibility offered by her body, Manheim has been trying to move away from the politicized position of fat acceptance spokesperson, a move that some critics have labeled disingenuous. "From here on out, I can just try to be the beautiful, sexy Camryn Manheim, but everyone's going to want to talk to me about it. I fear that the only way I'm going to get out from underneath the shroud of the torch carrier for fat acceptance is if I have something else I'm speaking out about, or I drop out of sight entirely, and that's what I plan to do."[38]

In answering the hypothetical question about what would happen if she lost weight, Manheim responds: "I'm not here to proclaim I love my body and I love being fat, I'm just here to say I love being myself. But if I choose to lose weight or find a way to lose weight that suits me, and doesn't make me feel deprived or angry or hostile, then I will do that. But you'll never catch me telling somebody about the pill I'm taking or the exercise routine I'm on, unless they inquire."[39]

Comedian and former talk-show host Rosie O'Donnell is also publicly talkative about her fatness and, as of this writing, has not reduced her weight to the point where she would be considered less than midsized. (Hard-line types might cast O'Donnell as something of a Traitor, given her promotion of the "eat less, move more" philosophy during her Chub Club years, but I consider her frequent presentation of antidiet rhetoric representative of an Out and About type. In a May 2001 interview on her show with singer Stevie Nicks, when Nicks spoke of hitting rock bottom at a weight of 170, Rosie chirped, "That's my goal weight!" While her comment sounds immediately like diet rhetoric, more than a moment's consideration reveals that her expressed ideal is a body weight much heavier than that expected of women these days.)

Representatives of Silent Types occupy public positions in their fat bodies but typically fail to acknowledge their size or the politics of fatness; however, they also fail to capitulate to self-hating diet rhetoric. Cohost of the daytime talk show *The View,* Star Jones, is an exemplar. Jones downplays her size as an issue;[40] she frequently sits in on interviews with entertainment-world beauties who fuss about diet tricks and exercise tips, but she never engages in rhetoric that would suggest that she thinks *she* should put these ideas to use. (Off camera, though, she has been known to reveal the truth about her model guests: "I've sat next to these cover models and thought to myself, 'Whoooo, girl, you're not looking so hot.' ")[41]

Members of the third category, Traitors, are those publicly fat individuals whose drastic dieting efforts or experience with weight-loss surgery front a devastatingly negative view of fatness. Prior to weight loss, some Traitors make a habit of publicly deriding their own bodies, while others declare comfort with their large size. Despite differences in their pre-weight-loss attitude, their dieting efforts and the rhetoric that accompanies them are implicated in what may be described as an attempt to "pass" in the world of "normal"-sized bodies. In her stand-up comedy act, Generation X spokesperson Janeane Garofalo jokes about Traitors, pointing out the significant number of celebrity women who betray their real-world counterparts by saying they love their bodies, only to slim down to unrecognizable proportions. Garofalo coyly jests, "I won't do that to you"; she's down with the cause, it seems. However, fans of the comic realize that her embrace of such a stance is ironic, given her frequent expressions of disdain for her more fleshy body parts (like the much-maligned back fat).

Excellent work on Traitors has been done by psychotherapists Beth Bernstein and Matilda St. John, whose focus on the "Roseanne Benedict Arnolds" examines how celebrity spokespeople betray fat women.[42] Bernstein and St. John discuss the cases of Ricki Lake, Carnie Wilson, Oprah Winfrey, and Roseanne as Traitors. For fat women, the most devastating of these turncoats is neither Lake nor Wilson, who are minor celebrities,[43] nor Winfrey, who has always disparaged her own fatness, but Arnold, whose anger, comic brilliance, and working-class sensibility came packaged in a self-appreciated body similar to the ones paraded by her fans. While Roseanne's autobiography claims her fat body as normal and comfortable, her public dieting and penchant for plastic surgery frame her as disappointingly hypocritical. Bernstein and St. John point out Arnold's contradictory impulses relative to fatness: "Only months after having her stomach reduced to the size of a thimble, Roseanne was vocal in her support of fat women: 'We're done with the skinny little victim girl thing. We love fat chicks on our show. A lot of the chicks watching are fat, too.' Sure, she loves fat chicks, but she will do anything not to be one of us, including a surgery that is, at its heart, self-mutilation."[44] While the authors concede that fat celebrities are not mandated to be fat advocates, they argue that because the celebrities use their body talk to build a fan base, their betrayals sting significantly.

The few celebrities who do out their own fatness provide role models for everyday folk who have begun to recognize the misfortune involved in passing as a thin-wannabe in a fat body. Writer and size acceptance activist Amy Walton hails the radicalism of outing unashamed fatness:

> Unrepentant fat girls are the real bad girls. Sexual lawlessness is so mainstream that we are selling it to teeny boppers. Think of how radical Girl Power would have been if the Spice Girls had all been fifty pounds heavier, ate grilled cheese sandwiches and french fries and still wore skimpy outfits—stomachs and cottage cheese thighs akimbo. Maybe that is what we need to break down the isolation of fat women. It's time to take fat out of the closet.[45]

Some have charged that fat can never really be closeted in the same way that sexuality can be, because of the obviously visual nature of fatness. Walton's comment illustrates how repentance about one's body forms a metaphorical closet for fat people, and urges us to imagine a world in which fat bodies are recognizable to one another without the patina of shame.

Fat activists regularly describe the experience of coming out as fat and choosing to no longer pass as on-the-way-to-thin. Back in 1983, Pam Hinden told what she called her "fat coming out story." She explained that coming out meant mustering courage to engage in activities usually thought proper only for thin people, giving up futile diets, and rebuilding her self-esteem.[46] She described being fat as the most intense experience of her life, more so than being Jewish, a lesbian, or even a woman. Such stories are common, and are described in greater detail in the next chapter.

Charlotte Cooper exhorts fat people to end their efforts to pass, arguing that they'll never be slim enough to be accepted and granted power and that meaningful social change for fat people as a group cannot occur when it is predicated on self-denial.[47] She underscores the value of coming out for fat people, or making public their otherwise discredited or invisible identities: "Although being out and open exposes me to potential ridicule, it also enables me to find allies in unexpected places. I do not want to live my life in fear, so instead of adopting a camouflage, I feel that it is more fruitful to develop assertive ways of protecting myself."[48]

Echoing the mantra of ACT-Up and Queer Nation, coming out as a fat person means announcing "We're here, we're spheres! Get used to it!"[49] While the command for *others* to get used to fatness rings loud and clear, fat people often manifest a sense of ambivalence about their own bodies. This may stem in part from their familiarity with the yoke of shame, but it is reinforced by the public expression of ambivalence about fat *by* fat people.

It is difficult for rank-and-file fat folk to embrace the idea that they're embraceable when their fat activist leaders express I'd-rather-be-thin sentiments. A *New York Times* article about diet-industry fraud testifies that Lynn McAfee, director of the Council on Size and Weight Discrimination, owns a product called the "Fat-Be-Gone ring," reputed (falsely) to utilize acupuncture principles to yield the same effect as jogging six miles a day. No, a declaration of high camp was not McAfee's intention. With some small shimmer of hope, she admits, "In the back of my mind, I say, Well, maybe it will work."[50] When this is the public declaration of a well-known fat advocate, the mind boggles at what the fat-*phobes* have in store. A reasonable public should allow their fat icons room for a little internal contradiction, but at what point does self-doubt become a self-defeating political strategy?

Even Nomy Lamm, fat feminist extraordinaire, expresses hard-toreconcile contradictions in her zine *I'm So Fucking Beautiful*. One moment, she warns those who fear her to "just wait," because the fat grrrl revolution has just begun. Then, without blinking, she gushes about a party where all the boys present said they had been attracted to her at some point.[51] Some fat people might expect a little more from their revolutionary icons than girlish giggling about being the object of someone's affection, however human that desire is. The apparent dilution of Lamm's punk attitude about fat oppression might be a function of the fact that she's explaining her zine to the readership of *Radiance*, a mainstream "big is beautiful" booster publication.

Internal contradictions about the meaning of fatness are nowhere more prevalent than in public figures attempting to gain mainstream credibility. Ricki Lake, *Hairspray* ingenue turned gab-show moderator, lost over a hundred pounds after accepting praise as a positive role model for young fat women. Her weight loss might be best explained if one considers her publicly announced aim: "My goal in life was to be loved and adored by everyone." Before the loss, she was adored by the size acceptance crowd, but apparently the adulation wasn't enough; instead, she starved herself to be accepted by mainstream America. She also claims, "I never set out to be a role model for large women."[52] This enforced dissociation is hard to swallow for legions of this former fat chick's fans.

What perhaps stings most is not the recognition that there are privileges associated with smaller body size, but that fat icons like Lake disavow any pleasure in fatness once they've lost weight. The guest editorial collective of the Canadian journal *Fireweed* articulates a position that suggests tolerance for ambivalence relative to fat pride. In discussing how their call for contributions led to a more diverse (and somewhat less fat-affirming) collection of writings than they had anticipated, they say: "We live a life of spreading the word on the beautiful world of big. We have a bevy of fat girl fans that follow our wide loads, and so we assumed that everyone's experience was relatively similar. What we forgot about in the sugar-hazed frenzy that brought us together, was the bad days. When nothing fits, including the chairs, and the most comfortable place to be is in bed."[53] A fat politics that fails to recognize the depressing aspects of oppression, and instead focuses on only the "positive" is doomed to fail.[54] McAfee needs space to covet the power generated by thin-privilege, but as a fat activist, she can work toward generating some privileges for her own cohort. Lamm would seem cartoonish and false if her brazen pro-fat attitude were not balanced by some small bit of concern about how others regard her. It is Lamm herself who has the last word on the usefulness of putting great faith in public icons to fight fat-liberation battles:

> While I spend day after day trying to get people to challenge their stereotypes and assumptions about fat people, I realize that I am a living replica of a popular stereotype: the fat, hairy, disabled Jewish dyke who is out to destroy the state. And you know what? That's a great thing to be. Let the Delta Burkes of the world break stereotypes by being corporate seductresses. I say: "Fine, I accept that I'm a freak. I'm a fat, sleazy, one-legged anarchist dyke, and I'm a total hottie."[55]

8

. . . .

The Resignification of Fat in Cyberspace

Judith Butler writes that "all social systems are vulnerable at their margins, and . . . all margins are accordingly considered dangerous."[1] The fat body, when read as disgusting, has been pushed to the margins of Western culture, but the resources of abjection there make the fat body, performed as subversive, quite threatening to comfortably held ideas about the social, political, and economic entitlement of those people currently ascribed as natural, beautiful, and healthy.[2] This chapter focuses on a community of bodies that have failed to materialize—that haven't been constructed as bodies—and examines their attempts to qualify as bodies that matter through the use of technology.

My primary purpose here is to investigate the embodied experience of fatness in spaces between subjectivity and subjection on various Internet newsgroups and lists. I examine how fat people are simultaneously constructed as *subjects* with the power to make choices about their bodies and the meanings written on their bodies (despite their choices being ultimately deemed "bad" or "unhealthy") and are *subjected to* fat oppression (or lack of will, depending on whom you ask). My ultimate goal in looking at the resignification of fat through technology is to change the terrain of relationships around fat, rather than to "celebrate or condemn particular political subjects."[3] My analysis will investigate the varied positions of agency of members of fat-related groups in an attempt to understand the contestatory nature of political struggle over—and social transformation of—the meaning of fat.

I am interested in investigating the Internet as a forum for political work, a "subaltern counterpublic"[4] that has the potential to create new rules for identity membership owing to the erasure of the physical on text-based sites. The context of the on-line communication about fat under investigation here is quite interesting historically: the two groups I examine, *FD* and *FAS*, have been around since not long after mainstream awareness of the Internet boomed with the information revolution of the early 1990s. *FAS* (discussions for anyone pro-fat) was founded in 1994 when a subset of users on a diet newsgroup splintered off into their own group after responding to self-loathing posts by talking about size acceptance, and *FD* (discussions about fat for pro-fat, pro-lesbian women) was founded in the summer of 1995.[5] (Interestingly, the *FAS* group was created by a user who was in favor of dieting for weight loss—so the new group served as a type of dungeon to which the fat-positive folks could be banished.) The conversations on both sites are set against a mainstream backdrop of contempt for fat, with public ridicule of fat people claimed by many to be the last socially-sanctioned-but-politically-incorrect form of humor. Diet and fitness industries are currently multibillion-dollar enterprises, and an estimated 20 to 40 percent of American adults are engaged in dieting behaviors, trying to make their fat disappear in favor of the slender, muscled body that is the choice signifier of health, beauty, and nature at the moment.[6]

The physical setting of the on-line discussion groups presents an invisible, text-only space for representing the fat body. My investigation is limited to an electronic list and a newsgroup, each of which is marked by the exchange of words, rather than pictures (with few exceptions). Members of the *FD* list belong to a moderated community, where the moderator functions mostly to screen out self-identified men and occasionally to remind subscribers of the group's charter. Participants on the *FAS* newsgroup may choose to indulge in or ignore postings from anyone, fat-positive or not, as the discussions are public. In one crucial difference between the groups, a large percentage of *FD* participants hail from the same large West Coast city, and often engage with one another in fat-related activities outside the list, while for most members of *FAS*, the newsgroup constitutes their only contact with like-minded others.

It is difficult to ascertain exactly how many people belong to each group, because of the possibility that a large number of participants prefer to simply read the postings of others rather than to post their own stories. Officially, according to the list wrangler, between two hundred and three hundred people subscribed to *FD* during my study. However, at any given time, the number of posting participants on *FD* might range from twenty to fifty, depending on level of interest in the topics being discussed at the moment. I have observed that following periods of intense conflict, when the number of daily postings increases dramatically, a significant number of participants deaffiliate from the list (though some of them return to the fold at a later time). Because the mechanics of a newsgroup are different from those of a list, with public postings and no subscription requirement, it is impossible to know how many silent participants there are. Still, on any given day, one can expect between fifteen and seventy-five posts on the *FAS* bulletin board.

While many of the members of both groups have been transient or silent over the years, each site has a core of dedicated participants, who must be noted for their ability to shape and sustain a large amount of fat-related conversation. Participants themselves on both sites have remarked that a large number of these key subscribers have graduate degrees and appear to work both early and late, judging by what they reveal about themselves and when they post.[7] Another set of individuals must be recognized as key players on both sites, though their contributions are neither frequent nor consistent: the provocateurs, or "flamers." These are people whose presence is usually short-lived and is marked by some sense of antagonism toward either the group in general or some perspective presented by one or more of the group members.

The two groups were established with slightly different mission statements, and thus the activities that occur on each site differ relative to the established boundaries. In both cases, though, the central activity is conversation that represents positive attitudes toward fat. These conversations take on any number of forms: from banter about where to buy speciality clothing and equipment, to discussions about the relationship of embodiment to sexuality, to exchanges of support for other participants facing discrimination from employers or medical doctors. Occasionally, the sites are used as advertising space for upcoming events of interest to many of the participants, like a fat women's swim night or a play party; of course, given the wide geographic dispersal of group members, such postings provide useful information to only a relatively small number of nearby participants. Still, the existence of such postings indicates the extent to which participants conceive of each other as "real" people who have lives apart from the computer screen. I believe that this recognition marks an interesting difference between discussion on these groups and the "hi, what are you wearing" conversations held on many other newsgroups and in chatrooms. In these fat groups, the participants often choose to reveal to one another their real names and even where they work, while in other cases they prefer to communicate using a coded user name. In any case, what is most important is connection to the other group members.

Because of the unique temporal character of on-line conversations, little things like clashing schedules don't get in the way of fat people connecting to one another. In the case of both groups, participants can read other postings whenever they desire and can post responses or start new conversational threads that will either be accessible for a few days on a public electronic bulletin board (in the case of *FAS*) or be delivered to the e-mail account of other list members (as in *FD*). My observations indicate that most participants, particularly those on *FD*, respond within hours (sometimes even minutes) to posts that interest them, thus preserving a sense of flow and continuity in the conversations. Postings to both sites happen at all times of the day and on every day of the week.

Because these sites are not communities in the traditional sense, and because their primary purpose is the sharing of self-posted information, there is little need to divide labor on the sites. On *FD*, the one person with a greater investment of time and labor than others is the list wrangler, who screens new subscribers for gender and who occasionally reminds the members of the list's mission statement, should controversy arise. The *FAS* group is run by an automated server, ensuring that anything that anyone posts will be made available on the bulletin board. On both sites, participants share responsibility for starting new threads and replying to others, but there are no serious consequences for failing to take these actions.[8]

It is important to discuss significant events occurring at these sites, along with their context and consequences. The events I will describe in this section stem from some of the continuing themes of discussion on either one or both sites: the "fit" of fat bodies within cyberspace versus in real space; guarding borders (both of the group and of fat identity); and strategies for resignifying fat.[9] The resulting interpretation of social rules and basic patterns of order on the sites should prove useful for understanding how communication at these sites both enables and constrains particular notions of fat identity.

Appreciation of the existence of on-line fat communities runs deep among both the users of *FD* and those of *FAS*, who often claim that they (both in identity and in physicality) do not "fit" in everyday encounters. One *FD* list member, when confronted with some intra-list squabbling about the sexual orientation of its members, put it this way: "I have yet to find any community that I fit into one-hundred-percent perfectly, and so when I find a community that most of me fits into, like this list, I get really concerned that I continue to mostly fit in."[10] Such a statement speaks not only to the vital social function of these communities, but also to the way in which users perceive themselves as outsiders of their regularly inhabited communities. Other users concur: "Thank goddess for this list; sometimes I feel like some kind of isolated freakozoid when I use how it feels to be out in the world as my only reality check," and "I realized that I don't know any lesbians who identify as fat dykes outside of my cyber-acquaintances on this list!"[11] One heated *FD* conflict about the male-oriented posts of heterosexual list members elicited this response, a plea for continued discussion in this place where fat women could finally fit comfortably: "I just really hate 'being where I'm uncomfortable' (a familiar theme to many of us, I assume, fat being a common denominator) and don't like to step on toes! I feel really good here."[12] (Although this excerpt sounds like it might have been a response to being personally targeted as "inappropriate," it was in fact posted by a member who had not been involved in the conflict until this moment.) The list is again praised as a comfort zone for women who don't seem to fit elsewhere.

Many posts outline important reasons for using the on-line space for communication: connecting with other fat women, lessening the social handicap of shyness, feeling empowered by the lack of immediate pressure to respond, and enjoying the "global village" effect. However, another reason cited for the appeal of on-line fat community space is the discomfort fat people often feel when congregating with one another in real space. For many, apprehension about being perceived as some type of pitiful spectacle keeps them isolated. One woman gave an example of such an instance: "My partner and I went on an all-gay cruise, and although 90% of the passengers were gay men, there were a dozen or so lesbians on board. Only one other couple were fat and they couldn't deal even being SEEN with another fat couple, let alone striking up a conversation with 'them' (us)."[13]

For some subscribers, it is the anonymity of cyberspace that is most attractive; the fact that they exist on-line only as words detached from their bodies frees them for less self-conscious reflection about the nature of their embodied experiences. "Although I'm new to this group, I'm sure it can go without saying that I've suffered abuse and humiliation as a life-long large female. I've never had the anonymity to be able to just blurt that out and I'm stunned at how sad it is to take suffering for granted just because of a body feature."[14] Other members point to the possibility that the on-line fat-community space provides a space for the airing of contradictions that might be used against fat people by unsympathetic others. In one post, an *FD* member praises the list for the diversity of perspectives it presents regarding fat acceptance, specifically in response to another member who said she wasn't as accepting of her own fat body as she would like to be.

> When people are just honest about where they are, while owning it as internalized oppression, what more can you ask? You won't make progress by pretending to be in some other place (not that I'm saying you are, but it seems that some folks want you to do that). And frankly that's what I think support groups (including this list) are *for*. You can't bring your fears and doubts and self-criticisms to the fat-phobes, they'd just say it proves their point. I think this is a great place for us to share the process of learning to love ourselves. . . . It's unfortunate that some people have no tolerance for anything less than perfect self-love. Hell, if we all had that, why would we even need a movement?[15]

This post invokes issues of internal strife over who is allowed to speak on the list and what they're allowed to say. For now, my focus is on the author's recognition of the list as a safe space for exposing the contradictions that can be used against fat people by people who don't share their perspective of fat acceptance.

Users on *FD* valorize the fat female form in cyberspace in other ways that mark them as outsiders from their communities. Frequently, their discussions of bodies and pleasures position fat women positively as active subjects of desire, encouraging them to take up much more space than they are usually considered to be entitled to:

> I've rarely been in the presence of another woman who physically overwhelms me, and that is something I would dearly love to experience. . . . That is usually an experience that comes in the presence of men. It's not the "maleness" of men that I fantasize about, but the physicality of them— height, breadth. . . . I do wish to have that feeling of being covered, surrounded, protected physically by another woman.[16]

Here, the on-line forum provides a place for the discursive affirmation of women whose bodies exert influence and take up space, an honor usually accorded to men.

Another reason participants value cyberspace, particularly in *FD*, is because it seems to provide a woman-only space so uncommon off-line. This gender parameter provokes significant discussion about the possibilities of organizing on-line from the borderlands of difference. One list member's anecdote about a "real world" experience of exclusion happened as the result of structural prohibitions against bisexuals and lesbians sharing the same floor at the annual Fat Women's Gathering on the West Coast. Her analysis of the event positions the *FD* list as an alternative space, large enough for everyone to participate in important conversations about fat.

> I remember there was a lesbian caucus meeting . . . and we had about 40 women. Next door there was supposedly a bi women's meeting, but as I recall, only 2 or 3 women showed up so they canceled it. That's *really* isolating, folks. I would not want to be a fat bi woman, looking for my community, and find that the only meeting for me was canceled and meanwhile, right next door, there's this huge meeting for fat women who love women, that I'm not allowed to go to. That sounds pretty damn depressing to me. Let's not let that happen again. I'd really like to see a more unified community. As fat women we don't have a lot of spaces in the world that are welcoming to us. Personally, I need all the allies I can get. And I sure don't want to make anyone feel isolated in the one place where they *should* feel they belong![17]

Here, the freedom of electronic space is contrasted with the restrictions of the way social and political organizations are frequently organized off-line: by identity, which is presumed to be singular. This demonstrates the ways in which boundaries from different domains manage to inform and shape one another.

If there is much at stake in deciding how identity is defined, there is also much at stake in choosing language to represent identities. Sometimes linguistic inventions can render identities intelligible even when their referents are ambiguous; take, for instance, the term *queer*, which *FD* members take to be a "generic term . . . which covers a multitude of sexualities."[18] Depending on how you look at it, *queer* may be a troubled term; some could argue that the term, and thus the identity, is colonized by people with very specific same-sex physical experiences, thus disallowing, say, a position of "straight queerness." This exclusivity arguably works to a political disadvantage for groups that might otherwise benefit from such surprises of diffuseness. Others might argue that when such a term is bandied about and self-applied liberally by those who otherwise suffer none of the plights of gays, lesbians, bisexuals, and transgendered people, it loses all meaning or is highly patronizing. One *FD* member suggests that "the term *queer* did have a distasteful sound to it in the 70s–80s . . . [but] now that the younger 'Gender Fuck' gays and lesbians use it all the time, it has started to be more and more accepted. It still pisses me off when other people say it, though, but it's cool when we use the term. Reclaiming our Queerness!"[19]

Using language to reclaim positive identity has been a project for fat communities as well. Many have campaigned for public acceptance of the term *fat* in place of euphemisms like "big-boned," "overweight," and "heavyset." One listmember claims that she is "conscious of this list removing the badness from the word *fat*. I use the word *fatdyke* from time to time and it shocks people and I think 'Yes!', go to work on your preconceived notions and biases!"[20] Still, nothing irks many fat people more than to hear a woman five pounds over life-insurance height-and-weight standards bemoan her personally and culturally imagined status as a "fat" person.[21] There is a sense on the sites that the term *fat* should be positively connoted but not watered down, not used to refer to bodies that really aren't fat. The question, is then, what does pass muster as an authentically fat body? How is it discursively constructed on-line, and need it strictly correlate with how the same body is materially constructed in the "real" world?

It is entirely possible that the fat bodies presented in these on-line sites could be total inventions, but admitting that does not strip them of their political volatility. In a language-only space, where nobody can see your hips, your belly, your legs, to say that you are fat is a strong, meaningful political gesture that says that fat will not be erased. Other than the narrative assertion "I am fat" with accompanying anecdotes about fat oppression suffered at the hands of fat haters (an important part of fat "credentialing" on these sites), there is just no simple way to be sure. A preoccupation with attaining certainty about "real world" body types diminishes the meaning taken from on-line performance. What *could be* becomes a much more interesting issue than what *is*, especially when "what *is*" is very much open to interpretation.

I am not trying to argue that these sites are purely creative zones where everyone just happens to love fat and where participants float around in bodies purchased with the currency of a few taps on the keyboard. Indeed, the space of the on-line fat body is maintained through the quelling of dissent and difference, mostly articulated by anti-fat flamers but sometimes voiced from within the groups.

In one instance, the occasion of internal dissent over appropriate minimum weight requirements on *FD* compelled some list members to reflect on the inherent relativity of *all* identities: "On that 200 lbs issue . . . if someone weighs 200 lbs, and is about . . . 4'10" or so . . . she is probably as fat as I am and faces the same issues . . . I still don't understand this arbitrary 200 lbs thingy . . . maybe we should have a height limit here . . . (sorry, I couldn't resist)."[22] This post gets at the difficulty of defining a real, essentially "fat" identity; not only is what is considered fat relative to a measure of height or other physical descriptors, as this author points out, but it is also relative to cultural standards and historical criteria.

One *FD* listmember summed up her sense of the utility of the list by saying that "you do what you can do and get by how you can. By creating supportive communities we work to accept ourselves, each other, and create change in the external world."[23] At this point I hope that I have made a strong case that on-line communication about fat identity and politics has the power to resituate users within discourse. Some may ask for "real" evidence, material indications that it's not all just "talk," that these on-line conversations do contribute to a large-scale, external resignification of fatness. In response, I can suggest a few examples of the small impacts that *FD* and *FAS* have had on the external world.

The first case deals with Fat Lip Readers Theatre, a Bay Area theater collective dedicated to the presentation of dramatic works that deal with issues of fat oppression. In April 1997, they posted to the *FD* list a notice that heralded a change in their organizational structure, a change perhaps modeled after the organizational structure of *FD* itself:

> Fat Lip has thus far been a closed group. . . . This will be changing. Instead we will have a central group of women . . . which will guide the activities of the group, but the general membership of the group will be fluid, allowing interested women to participate on a project-to-project basis. . . . Fat Lip will continue to be for fat women only, but we'll continue to work with other size acceptance groups to strengthen our community. [The central group, known as "the Hub"] has come up with a mission statement: "The Hub is a coalition dedicated to increasing the visibility and availability of size positive activities, resources, and organizations in the greater San Francisco Bay Area."[24]

What I find most compelling about this is the move away from organization based on shared essential traits, toward affinities of action. While there is still some identity-based core, the new emphasis is on working with others to achieve similar goals.

Other fat groups around the country borrow the cultural agitation tactics of the Lesbian Avengers, preferring spectacularly staged events to boring political rallies as a means of exhibiting their subjectivity.[25] Frequently, users post notices about events such as a group scale-smashing under Seattle's Space Needle, a collective scale toss from the Golden Gate Bridge, a "No Diet Day" bookmarking in a large New York City bookstore's self-help section, and even an ice cream eat-in on the front lawn of a busy Boston Jenny Craig diet center. Another fun form of direct action, possible from the comfort of one's own living room, involves applying "Feed This Woman" stickers onto ads featuring very thin models and sending the ads back to the companies.[26] Judging from the on-line discussion of these types of events both before and after, the fat site users aren't just a damp bunch of pasty-skinned computer geeks whose only light is the flicker of their monitors; they're as physically active and bold (and, of course, sometimes as couch-potatoey and mild) as they are online. Their subversion of mainstream standards of acceptable physicality is small, dispersed, and local, but it is exactly this kind of subversion that provides the best (because most radically democratic) opportunities for reimagining what counts as healthy and beautiful.

To sum up, fatness can be reconfigured from a spoiled identity to a proudly inhabited one by using any number of strategies aimed at entering fat bodies into discourse proudly and publicly. This task, though, is never easy and is very risky. One *FD* listmember who has been at it for years says, "It takes all of my strength every damn day to get out there and be myself, stay centered in my being, come across as the woman I truly feel myself to be and not think about or take in people's negative response to my physical being."[27] Still, the sense I get from the two groups is that the possibility of resignifying fat—of finally (though partially) inhabiting the position of "subject" rather than constantly "subjugated"—is well worth the effort and the risk.

I have tried to pay particular attention to the contradictions inherent in the conversations on-line. Mara Math, an *FD* listmember, talked about the will to innocence that one encounters in most groups that are striving to invigorate their individual subject positions:

> My experience has been that every movement has its excesses around the cusp of first gaining power. Remember the days when the line was that all lesbian sex was perfect? As were all lesbian relationships? (And there are often far crueler excesses as well.) I suspect that this rush-of-power/reverse of the pendulum re. Fat Lib takes the same route: fat is unequivocally good, and absolutely the only thing wrong is social oppression. I think paying attention to these contradictions (without yielding to oppressive bullshit) would serve us well.[28]

This chapter, then, is intended to place those contradictions under a magnifying glass in an effort to debunk the strategic efficacy of innocence in favor of a more complex scheme for recognizing the contested character of fat identity. Elizabeth Grosz recognizes that the realization that "one's struggles are inherently *impure*, bound up with what one struggles against" is troubling, in that it "refuses the idea of a space beyond or outside, the fantasy of a position insulated from what it criticizes and disdains."[29] We see complicity happening in cyberspace: those seeking to reconfigure the fat body *must*, to some degree, work in tandem with the kinds of ideas and ideal bodies they are trying to destroy.

Patricia Mann writes that "those of us who are not physically assimilable stand upon previously unremarked boundaries of liberal universalism, representing its de facto exclusionary capacities for all to see" but also assures us that "it is [our] . . . visible physical markings . . . that allow us to represent our political agency most vividly."[30] Though the spaces I have examined in this chapter are text-based, they work to represent a politicized surface for the fat body. It is remarkably apparent from posts like the last one that the on-line groups can provide a steady anchoring point, as well as a point of departure, for fat subjectivity.

In *Gender Trouble*, Judith Butler argues that the body's surface is politically constructed.[31] While her focus is on issues of sex/gender construction, my efforts are directed at denaturalizing and resignifying categories of body size and shape. Butler accomplishes her task by highlighting the subversive potential of parodic practices, which certainly find their parallels in fat politics in the guise of events like fat lingerie shows and fat Star Trek conventions, campier even than the draggiest drag. Though in these on-line sites there is not such a strong visual sense of parody, users have indeed appropriated and reworked vocabularies and symbols from the dominant mainstream to their own advantage; the prevalence of the word *fat* in the movement, instead of euphemisms like *heavy-set,* is a case in point.

Butler points to other areas where "discourse reiterate[s] injury such that the various efforts to recontextualize and resignify a given term meet their limit in this other, more brutal, and relentless form of repetition," citing the success of reworking *queer* and the failure of reappropriating *nigger.*[32] I believe that a resignification of "fat" is poised somewhere in between these two; in some kind of aural slide, being called "phat" is the freshest form of flattery, but it's still disconcerting to be told you're looking chunky.[33] The comfort with which on-line participants freely use *fat* to describe themselves positively is still challenged by the brutally negative cultural repetitions of the adjective as a put-down.

It appears that the strategies mobilized on-line in the instances I have examined allow fat people to claim their subjectivity, while they slowly and unevenly rework the rules of what counts as healthy and beautiful. The participants assume the position of the speaking subject within their on-line language communities, providing a frame of reference for their citation as healthy and beautiful within the larger language communities in which they operate. The strengths of the groups are their flexibility and continuing dedication to discussing the difficulties of pragmatic struggle over the resignification of fat.

These conversations are effective forms of political action. Butler claims that power relations both constrain and constitute the very possibilities of volition; one cannot withdraw or refuse power, only redeploy it.[34] While I don't imagine that a bunch of fat people sitting in front of their computers typing away is likely to be read as an attempted coup or as a transcendence of oppressive relations around body size and shape toward limitless pleasure in the fat body, I would argue that the conversations they engage in do subversively redeploy a sense of entitlement about the possibilities of taking pleasure in and by fat bodies. They have no plans for some fat separatist utopia; instead, their power is more what Butler describes as

> a kind of diffuse corporeal agency generated from a number of different centers of power. Indeed, the source of personal and political agency comes not from within the individual, but in and through the complex cultural exchanges among bodies in which identity itself is ever-shifting, indeed where identity itself is constructed, disintegrated, and recirculated only within the context of a dynamic field of cultural relations.[35]

She argues for "the production of new subject-positions, new political signifiers, and new linkages to become the rallying points for politicization."[36] Although fat site users rarely explicitly indicate their intentions, the project of their discussions is to revamp their subjectivities, accord new usefulness to the signifier of fat, and to explore new linkages of affinity and action. As I have shown, they squabble all the way through these processes, but their factionalization does not produce political paralysis. Indeed, I want to plumb their sense of *dis*identification with one another for its political merits. As Butler claims, "the affirmation of that slippage, that failure of identification is itself the point of departure for a more democratizing affirmation of internal difference."[37]

What is vital is that users not let their squabbling get in the way of their continued self-signification, so essential to future possibilities for citing fat as healthy and beautiful and powerful. Curiously, members keep talking to one another; in a move reminiscent of Butler's "double movement," they "invoke the category [of fatness] and, hence, provisionally . . . institute an identity and at the same time . . . open the category as a site of permanent political contest."[38] Though users utilize identity terms with almost every utterance, they also constantly question them.

9

. . . .

Fat Politics and the Will to Innocence

Low self-esteem, my ass. Get your fucking foot off my neck.
FD user signature

Security is merely a superstition. It does not exist in nature nor
do the children of woman as a whole experience it. Security in the
long run is no safer than outright exposure. Life is a daring ad-
venture or nothing at all.
Attributed to Helen Keller by an FD user signature

When one considers the preponderance of anti-fat propaganda in circulation, it is difficult to criticize the choices that assimilationist fat activists
make in response. Public discourse generally suggests that fat people are
victims of their own undoing. A website featuring standard "your
momma . . ." jokes lists its fat jokes under the heading of "hygiene" rather
than "body type," a decision that reveals underlying assumptions about
the perception of culpability relative to fatness.[1] According to this logic,
an individual is fully responsible for the care and cleaning of his or her
own body, but can rarely do much about his or her natural somatotype.

"Your momma" fat jokes are small potatoes compared to the more
virulent anti-fat assertions of those who have the ear of the public. Rid-
iculing a fat activist who proclaims that fat people are on the march for
rights in record numbers, *American Spectator* writer Mark Steyn simpers,
"If only. Alas, she was speaking metaphorically. But fat people are on the
drive, wedged behind the steering wheel with a couple of Twinkies for

the road and heading straight for the latest fat rights demo, with a quick stop at the drive-thru Dunkin' Donuts."[2] Certainly, Steyn's inflammatory rhetoric warrants some response; but beware the impulse to saint fat people in order to protect them from the barbs of Steyn and his compatriots.

Fat activists of the assimilationist stripe typically respond to such charges by deploying a rhetoric of innocence which seeks to relieve them of responsibility for their much maligned condition. One example is the way innocence has been professionally mobilized in the hypothesizing of a pair of psychologists. With the intention of changing fat-phobic views, they argued that if fat women accessed information indicating they were blameless for being fat, then they would engender more positive attitudes toward fat people generally and themselves in particular.[3]

The will to innocence manifests itself in a variety of ways in the rhetoric of the size acceptance movement. Frequently advanced are links between fatness and low socioeconomic status that result in an inability to afford healthy food, which further exacerbates fatness. Also popular is patronizing portraiture of fat people (especially racial/ethnic minority members) as ignorant of proper nutrition and thus potentially salvageable should they become enlightened. Some arguments, though, depend on the logic that fat people should not be held responsible for their bodies because they don't eat any more than thin people do. Other tactics include moral segregation of the "fit" fat from the general fat population and the deployment of fatness as an inexplicable and uncontrollable condition.

One of the most subtle is the method of praising fat fitness overachievers and suggesting that despite their girth, they deserve to be treated well because their deeds make them healthy. Studies done at the Cooper Institute of Aerobics Research in Dallas indicate that nearly half of obese men have no increased mortality rate.[4] In other words, they're just as healthy as thinner men. Referring to a triathlete with a body mass index of 40 (which is well into obesity territory), a scientist at the Cooper Institute said, "I am confident that there are many obese people out there who are eating a healthy diet, who exercise regularly, who don't smoke but who are still fat. I say, lay off these people."[5] Though it is reassuring that "responsible" fat people may be given some leeway by this pronouncement, what about the rest of us non-triathletes? Only some fat people—the athletic types—are granted freedom from the harassment of subjugation in this scheme.

The notion that the great unwashed masses are largely ignorant about proper nutrition also circulates freely within public discourse. *New York Times* reporter Gina Kolata, in part of a bloated series on "the obesity epidemic," tells of the surprise expressed by Mexican American participants in an experimental diet program, who discovered that foods they habitually ate received a nutritional red light. "Esther Castro Rodriguez . . . said she was reeling after learning that peanut butter was in the red category. 'I thought that because it was vegetable oil it was good,' Mrs. Rodriguez said."[6]

A related *Times* piece describes a Howard University-based program called the "Cardiovascular Risk Factor Reduction Project," also known as "the obesity project," that is aimed at teaching African Americans "how to get healthy by eating right, exercising, and, not so incidentally, losing weight."[7] Author Natalie Angier emphasizes that industrialized nations now recognize thinness as a sign of status and education: "It was the most educated sector of the population that learned first about the benefits of fruits, vegetables and whole grains over such American staples as meat, milk and Wonder Bread."[8] How wickedly lovely to think that fatness will just go away once the Latinos and blacks learn how to eat right: isn't this implied by the *Times* pieces? This faulty perspective suggests that the reason people are fat is because they are ignorant, an especially insulting conclusion. It turns a blind eye to those fat people— most of us, even, who have had a lifetime of experience with food pyramids, puny serving sizes, and live-healthy diet sermons—who do indeed know what food is fattening and eat it anyway.

Even when public discourse concedes that fat people might actually understand concepts of proper nutrition, they are "saved" by the notion that their low socioeconomic status makes them financially unable to afford healthy provisions. Angier cites a series of studies by Drs. Anne Ellaway and Sally Macintyre of the MRC Medical Sociology Unit in Glasgow, Scotland, who found that "in low-income neighborhoods of Edinburg, items like whole-grain bread, fruits, vegetables and skim milk were not only more expensive than less-healthful items like packaged white bread and sausages, they were also more expensive than comparable healthful items for sale in high-income neighborhoods. In addition, the quality of produce in low-income shops was decidedly inferior to that in upper-income neighborhoods."[9] Safely out of their own control, the fat poor are thus freed of having any responsibility for their reviled state.

Unfortunately, though, their moral protection is founded on a loss of political control as well.

Another manifestation of the will to innocence comes in the form of reactionary arguments that fat people eat no more than thin or average-sized people.[10] While I understand the impulse to contravene declarations that fat folk are voracious, eating-obsessed pigs with this statement of empirical fact, I believe that allowing oneself to engage in such a debate drains pro-fatness rhetoric of its power. Saying "I don't eat any more than anyone else" basically says, "I can't help it—I'm not fat because of anything I did—so leave me alone." It also says, "I will allow my right to exist as a subject (reflective, reasonable, with power to act) to be predicated upon how much I eat or don't eat"—and this is ultimately a self-defeating move.

Other stories appropriated to support fat acceptance position fatness as inexplicable and beyond the control of the individual. In her research on weight-based discrimination, attorney Sondra Solovay marshals the complicated narrative of Christina and Marlene Corrigan to demonstrate what she calls "fat bias" in the pursuit of justice.[11] Christina died at age thirteen weighing 680 pounds; her mother, Marlene, was charged with felony child abuse/neglect. Apparently, Christina had experienced seizures as a baby and was treated with barbituates that slowed her metabolism; she gained weight rapidly throughout her childhood, despite "normal" eating habits. Basic tests showed nothing wrong with her, but she suffered humiliation in medical offices and while attempting to maneuver around her public school. Christina, who had not been feeling well, died while her mother ran out to the store; her body was found on the floor, covered with feces and bedsores, surrounded by fast food wrappers.

While one might imagine that the condition of Christina's body was cause for legal concern, the deputy district attorney in the case seemed to be motivated more by a sense of disgust about her fatness: "It was widely reported that overfeeding and 'allowing' Christina's weight gain were factors."[12] Solovay points out that no investigation was made into the difficulty of preventing bedsores for a 680-pound housebound body or the possibility that the feces were the result of the body voiding at death, and highlights the inefficacy of the autopsy that was performed on Christina. Although the cause of Christina's death did not imply neglect by her mother, Marlene was nonetheless found guilty of a misdemeanor.

Because of the ambiguity surrounding the cause of Christina's death, this is a difficult case to use to exemplify anti-fat bias. When resuscitating Marlene's character as loving and concerned, the tendency is to emphasize the uncontrollable nature of Christina's fatness. This is problematic because mobilizing a movement from a "poster child" mentality (à la Jerry's kids, suffering, pathetic, at the mercy of larger forces) tends to foster pity more than anything, and fails to position its members as subjects with the means to act upon the world. In her treatment of weight-related discrimination, Solovay relies heavily on cases where children and/or babies are inexplicably fat, prone to massive weight gain in short periods of time—suggesting that one must exonerate these "victims" from control over their own bodies before one can sympathize with their oppression. Only by reframing the "moral weakness" of fatness as a medical problem do many fat activists see hope. In fairness to Solovay, she does admit that "for some fat people, weight is mutable"[13] but also argues that this small percentage should not interfere with protection from discrimination for the rest. I want to flip this logic on its head and suggest instead that just because weight is immutable for some doesn't mean they have an exclusive claim ticket on protection from discrimination. Even if one does bring on one's own bodily state of fatness, that shouldn't preclude one's protection from discrimination, from the opportunity to live a happy and full life.

In spite of a history of being sniped at by medical representatives of the scientific establishment, many size-acceptance activists embrace scientific rhetoric to counter mainstream assumptions about the unhealthiness and lack of willpower of fat people, as well as successfulness of diets. They choose this route because the alternative seems to be agreement that fat is always unhealthy, fat folk are always weak-willed, and diets always work if the dieter just tries hard enough. But embracing the rhetoric of science is not the most advisable means of avoiding the absolutes of fat-hatred; such a strategy upholds the validity of judgments made by an external authority (in this case, science/medicine) to resuscitate one's character.

On the grounds that the studies are biased by financial motivations, critics repudiate scientific studies that conclude that dieting is a successful enterprise. They counter "bad" science with what they describe as more "objective" and "good" science. In her study of fat-oriented publications, Leslie Haravon admits that "while there are many diet scams that thrive without the verification of medical professionals, anti-diet movements would be utterly unsuccessful without such scientific backing."[14] She makes similar claims about the necessity of employing scientific "counterfacts" to disrupt the mythic concept that fat is unhealthy. Likewise, assertions that fat people are weak-willed and out of control are renounced by recourse to arguments about body size and diet-breaking behavior as biologically "normal" or genetically motivated. The master's tools of medical fact seem unable to dismantle the house of fat oppression built on a foundation of scientific rhetoric.

Rather than presenting scientific counterfacts to propel fat acceptance, activists might do well to embrace the contradictions of the lived experience of fatness. That involves recognizing that sometimes fat is healthy, and sometimes it's not; that every person, fat and thin alike, has moments of self-control to parallel their times of abandon; and that diets do work sometimes, though the choices one makes in order to achieve considerable weight loss frequently reduce one's quality of life. Pro-fat protesters can challenge received knowledge using these contradictions as a start but will ultimately prove more effective at redefining fat identity if they create new paradigms for thought instead.

The will to innocence is futile as a political strategy, for while it makes fat people more sympathetic, it also paints them as incompetent and powerless. Statistics from the National Center for Health Statistics indicate that poor and less well educated adults tend to be fatter than their wealthier and better-educated counterparts.[15] Nonetheless, to embrace "I can't afford good food," "I never learned to eat properly," or "I have no control over my own body" as a self-preservationist salvo is wrongheaded on multiple counts. First, to do so is to perpetuate the search for a cause or an explanation for fatness, whereas no parallel search exists for bodily "normalcy"; second, to argue such points is to disavow one's own corporeal agency, a dangerous strategy for those who seek their long-awaited day in the sun of subjectivity.

Although I do not endorse the will to innocence as a political tool for redefining fatness, I recognize the reasons for its popularity. Take the case of Toni Cassista, a California woman who sued her employer, a food collective, for discriminating based on the perception that her fatness was disabling, when in fact it was not. Cassista lost, but others who sued, arguing that they were in fact disabled, won.[16] Though the Americans with Disabilities Act protects individuals who are *not* disabled but are mistakenly perceived to be, our cultural climate seems to mandate that only those who cast themselves in the role of victim (of real physical "injury," not just bad vibes) be given their due.[17]

Fat is treated as volitional—"a choice made out of laziness, hostility, social disdain, or other moral shortcomings like lack of willpower, failure of motivation, greed and dependence"[18]—so the tendency when dealing with this regressive attitude is to suggest that fatness cannot be helped. I wonder what would happen if, instead of giving up our volition, we worked to alter the terms of the choice, to emphasize that subjectivity mustn't be predicated on perception of innocence. Feminist theoretical underpinnings for abandoning the will to innocence found in the work of Judith Butler and Donna Haraway will be useful to future generations of fat activists, who will benefit from recognizing that innocent origins and unified identity need not undergird political struggles.[19]

Wendy Chapkis, decrying a political return to biological determinism as a guarantor of civil rights protection, reminds us that "difference may arguably be described as a 'fact of nature,' but its expression remains a social and political act. That right to enact difference—without relinquishing human and civil rights—can only be collectively won or lost, not partially extended on a case by case basis to those considered deserving by 'the rest of us.' "[20] Note the obvious parallel here to religion. Some of us choose our religion, some are born to it and never change, but all religious freedoms are afforded nonetheless. One of the major tasks facing fat activists is to ensure widespread public recognition that fatness is a state marked by internal contradictions that nonetheless warrants subjectivity.

A few brave souls already tread this path, like fat activist Marilyn Wann. In response to the charge that fat people are out of control, instead of downplaying her own agency, Wann enjoins fat folk to really get out of control, suggesting that they've been terribly dormant too long.

> If we *were* out of control, every time someone made some nasty comment about weight, we'd just sit on them until they apologized. If we got really good and out of control, we'd boycott the diet industry and show them who's boss. We'd run amok with chainsaws, whacking out the armrests in movie theaters and commercial airliners. We'd stage sit-ins at New York fashion shows, in state legislatures, on beaches. . . . Fat people out of control? I can't wait![21]

T. J. Bryan also offers a counterpoint to the will to innocence, claiming:

I'm fat, but I ain't no fuckin' saint. Middle-of-the-way membership has its
perks. An intimate inmate on the outskirts of massivity and magacentricity
simultaneously, I fearfully envision same-life Karmic repercussions, punishment incurred by my own actions and words. The first to dismiss political
propriety when pissed, I'm dangerously aware. Knowing better. Knowing
all too well where and how it hurts.[22]

"Middle-of-the-way membership" resonates with accepting the contradictions of fatness and disavowing the impulse to save oneself via recourse
to innocence. Bryan does note that her refusal to let herself off the hook
for her body may incur punishment but still prefers the option of using
power when she needs to.

Further questioning the wisdom of fat sainthood is the work of British
activist Charlotte Cooper. "Fat people have as much right to be greedy,
lazy, unfit or smelly as thinner people. By wanting to present only what
we feel is positive and acceptable," we are unfairly and unnecessarily
limiting ourselves.[23] Genteel types are likely to raise an eyebrow at this,
asking why anyone would strive for what seems like a compromised re-
ception rather than a more heraldic, celebratory understanding of themselves. When faced with invisibility, freaks "often prefer the risk and
blame associated with an intensely marked body and identity to the dis-
regard and neglect . . . of bourgeois Anglo-American culture."[24] If fat activists can muster the courage to take the risk of letting their freak status
show, the political payoff is promising.

My readings of discourse in fat-related cyberspace suggest that although users have made strides away from purely optimistic visions of
diet-free, fat-favoring "chubtopia," there still exists evidence of longing
for secure identities. I recall an interesting April 1997 FD posting in which
the author, raving about her attendance at the Michigan Wimmin's Music
Festival, encourages others to go, commanding them to "prepare to have
your eyes opened and to learn about our culture as lesbians. . . . Imagine,
an entire week with no contact from male dominated society!" While the
author's enthusiasm about throwing off the chains of male-dominated
society is admirable, it is hard for me to imagine that lesbians, even those
who've trekked to Michigan to hear good music, are no longer part of
male-dominated society, simply by virtue of being there and being queer.
To the author, I might say "Get used to it!"—the "it" being the continuing struggle one faces to validate one's identity and practices in fields of
power marked by constant fluctuation. (At the same time, though, I would

ask what kinds of validations *have* been successfully effected, in terms of preconceptions of straight, bi, and gay worlds.) The same goes for fat activists, who should not expect that all their work to change the cultural meaning of fat will someday provide them with a cushy pedestal upon which to permanently recline and revel in the glory of their newly fabulous double chins. This is diet mentality. There will be no security, even after a prolonged period of struggle; constant playfulness, maintenance, and vigilance will be necessary.

Indeed, there is no security in the explanations one holds for the existence of fat bodies; battles between nature and nurture loom large and stand little chance of being resolved anytime soon. One *FD* user suggests that to feel "safe," one should cultivate a healthy tolerance for ambiguity in such issues: "I wish that the 'we are born this way' people would realize that individuals may have a different life experience, and the 'we choose this' people would realize that for some of us, the only choice is between misery and being ourselves."[25] This member recommends staying alert for meanings different from one's own rather than resting comfortably on the laurels of easy subjectivity or simplified subjection.

Other list members assess which vision of fatness—subjectivity or subjection—is more useful in reconfiguring cultural meanings for fat. In the domain of health and medicine, fat has already undergone a transformation in some minds because many researchers now believe in the existence of a fat gene to which people are subjected, rather than mere laziness, compulsive eating habits, and lack of individual will as the cause of fatness. But is this transformation a useful one for fat people?

> Biological determinism is a hazardous way to try to get our rights. First, medicine has often in history been twisted and used as support for discrimination against groups of people. (I grew up thinking women could never have important jobs because our hormones were uncontrollable and our brains were too small.). . . . I certainly think there are many people who do not have reasonable choices about their size or sexual preference, but many of us do. Even if I didn't think I had a choice, I would hate to be characterized as a victim of my biology, an object of pity for others who are more "in control" of their biology. Fat people have recently been moved from the category of "morally inferior" to "biologically inferior" by the recent research discoveries. I don't think this move has helped us; if anything, there's more of an effort to "fix" our bodies at any cost.[26]

Here the author points to the idea that even cultural transformations that seem intended to destigmatize can position their constituents in politically precarious places. Thus, one must accept etiological ambiguity and resist the temptation to affix a cause, even an apparently forgiving one, to the health condition of fatness—in other words, stop asking "why?" about fat identity, and start acting out about it. Many members don't like "no-choice" explanations for both fatness and sexuality because, as they argue convincingly, "There should be size-acceptance and queer rights whether or not we have a choice about being fat or queer."[27] Others respond in a personally compelling manner, saying, "If it seems like it helps 'the cause' (or just saves my butt) I will assert that I 'can't help' being a lesbian. I think we can and should lie to people if it keeps us from getting bashed or discriminated against."[28] Being watchful over politicized meanings requires conceding that, theories aside, fat and queer people do get bashed and need strategies for dealing with that reality other than a pie-in-the-sky consolation that they have the power to rewrite the script of fat.[29]

Fat people have to be like the sexual subjects discussed by Elizabeth Grosz—both "subjects and deprived of a socially recognized subjective position . . . and beings who have a sexuality, but whose sexual specificities are ignored, denied, or covered over"[30]—for fat politics to make any sense at all. It is clear that an increasingly large number of fat-positive participants recognize their involvement in redefining fatness as part of a larger political movement aimed at just such ends. This recognition entails a sense of the history of identity-based movements:

> Maybe the "born this way" approach, where the trait in question is seen as something you can't control, is necessary in the beginning of a movement, when the people involved are just beginning to politicize the issue from a previous, pathologizing view. There's a journey that people have to take, where at first they're buying into the culture's view of pathology, and then they're willing to look at the possibility that they're really ok and it's the culture that's screwed up. But even there, they still have to deal with a lot of internalized shame. It takes a while to get that out of one's system. And I think that's where the idea of "we can't help it" is appealing. It's a bridge—a very useful bridge—in the process of going from internalized shame to acceptance, then on to turning it back outward and working toward making change in society (not that both processes can't overlap).
>
>   I think that when a group of people have attained a more secure place in society (relative to where they were before, that is), there is less need, at least internally, for people to convince themselves they're ok by saying it's not their fault and they can't help it. Once you actually believe a trait is ok, then why do you need to believe you can't help yourself? It becomes ok to choose it at that point.

Since the truth is—for both sexuality and body size—that there are elements of both biological determination *and* choice involved (over the population as a whole, not necessarily for each individual), it's not as though the movement is making the "inborn" argument up out of whole cloth. The "inborn" aspect of fatness or gayness is true—it's just not the whole truth. But it's possible to shade the truth this way or that, to suit the current need. As the movement matures, and more members begin to feel positive about who they are, then it becomes easier for the movement to incorporate into its position that yes, some of its members *have* made choices that have given them their identity of queer or fat.[31]

While this discussion-list member focuses specifically on the question of choice as it concerns identities, I think her comments are salient for helping to understand where many fat-positive individuals conceive of themselves as existing politically. Her commentary reflects a fascinating mixture of theoretical vocabulary, New Age expressions, and sophisticated lay interpretation of scientific dilemmas, a fusion of the discourses that constitute the faces of many identity-based groups struggling to strengthen their subject position.

Grosz claims that "for the subject to take up a position as a subject, he must be able to situate himself as a being located in the space occupied by his body. This anchoring of subjectivity in *its* body is the condition of coherent identity."[32] Throughout this book, I have provided multiple examples of ways in which fat-positive public discourse provides such a steady anchoring point, as well as a point of departure, for fat subjectivity, even when mitigated by the allure of being "let off the hook" for one's own deviance.

Indeed, the resignification process is not an all-or-nothing enterprise, as my personal experience demonstrates. I have been struggling for almost ten years to retrain myself in the ways I think about, appreciate, and respond to fat bodies. This effort began, strangely enough, not when I was fat, but just after I had lost a hundred pounds and was concerned that my weight loss would be read (against my intentions) as "finally taking care of myself," "getting a body to match that pretty face," "overcoming my need for protection from my sexuality," or any of the other host of "compliments" people pay those who successfully lose a considerable amount of weight. Since then, I've used every opportunity imaginable to publicly appreciate fatness, whether that means sincerely complimenting a fat stranger who has been bold enough to wear a bikini on the beach, stump-speeching my friends who whine as if it's the end of the world because they are having a "fat day," not fretting if I myself gain weight, or enjoying and circulating zines like *FaT GiRL*. Professionally, I have written for several years on strategies for repositioning the fat body as healthy and powerful.

This is not merely a pro-fat "facade" hiding a fat-phobic interior, but a complicated performance capable of being interrupted, as it was a few years ago. As I was strolling with a friend of mine, discussing the upcoming publication of my coedited anthology on the power and politics of corpulence, I mentioned that my coeditor would be moving away soon. My friend asked, "Is she fat, too?" Before I could respond, he quickly fumbled and said, "Not that you're fat, I mean, you're not, I don't know why I said *too*. Sorry. Because I don't think that you are . . ." It was a moment of genuine internal contradiction for me. On one plane, I felt surprised that he would apologize to me for implying that I was fat, given that my scholarly work was so strongly geared toward repositioning fat as fabulous. (What's wrong with being fabulous, after all?) At the same time, I recognized the grip that the mainstream signification of fatness seemed to have on him, and I felt strangely complimented by his revision of his own remark, positioning me as *not* that bad, out-of-control thing that a fat woman is supposed to be. Then, Catholic upbringing firmly in tow, I was riddled with guilt for feeling relieved that I had "passed" as not fat in this situation.[33] Of course, I also wondered if indeed he *did* think me to be fat, but normative forces of politeness had kept him from fessing up to this faux pas. I simply responded, "Yes, she is fat, and whether or not you think *I* am, it doesn't insult me. I have evolved." The point is this: Even with all my consciousness, I got caught up in that moment in negotiating the many layers of contradiction and expression happening so fleetingly, and in trying not to be hurt, once again, by being called a name, by being called fat.

In seeking to avoid such injury, I, as a being who requires language in order to be, defer to the power of language. Judith Butler claims that "we are vulnerable to language because we are constituted within its terms."[34] Though being called a name can hurt, it is also a moment of possibility for countering the offense, in that being called a name (interpellated) is one of the necessary moments in constituting a subject in language.[35] I have utilized my feelings of injury because of how I have been called to examine the terms of that address. In a related vein, even if my own work on the (previously invisible) fat subject within scholarly circles fails to address fat subjectivity in all of its compelling moments, and even if my interpretations are a bit "off" at times, my project does call fat subjects to action and gives them a point of departure for articulating themselves. If we exist by virtue of a "fundamental dependency on the address of the Other," then it is vital to be addressable and addressed.[36] Because language has the power to both sustain and threaten the body's existence, it is important to be properly engaged in language games about fat to stave off the threats and to concentrate efforts on sustenance.

The goal of fat-positive discourse, that which finally allows fat to come out on top, does imply the continued presence of a hierarchy of bodies, with a somewhat different ordering. While I believe this to be a commonly perceived outcome of the resignification of fatness, I would like to instead substitute Butler's notion of radical democracy wherein seemingly necessitated political signifiers are perpetually rearticulated in relation to one another, thus abandoning the revolving totem pole model of subjectivity. She argues for "the production of new subject-positions, new political signifiers, and new linkages to become the rallying points for politicization,"[37] and while fat-positive discourse rarely comes with a user manual that explains individual intentions, its overarching aim is to revamp fat subjectivity, accord new usefulness to the signifier of fat, and to explore new linkages of affinity and action.

There is a growing body of critical literature aimed at outlining the regulatory practices within which bodily forms are fabricated, to which I believe this book contributes an investigation of the ways in which negotiating questions of fat identity involves a fluid, alternating pattern of invocation and refusal of mainstream tropes of health, nature, and beauty. My goal has been the analysis of and critical intervention in the rules and practices guiding the entrance of the fat subject into discursive agency.

In my thematization of fat-positive public discourse, I have located repetitive, local strategies for subverting and contesting conceptions of fat as abnormal and for negotiating a livable fat subjectivity. Much as the rank and file are making themselves citable as healthy and beautiful through language, I want this book to be citable, a piece of scholarship to which future positive significations of fat can refer, as my own work refers to the earlier efforts of amazing groups like the Fat Underground. However, I realize that it is impossible to completely master the trajectory of anything you enter into discourse; it's a risky enterprise, in that just as terms have been turned against you in the past, so they can be in the future. But to echo Butler's sentiment on taking the risk,[38] we are politically compelled to claim fat and do what we can with it, because it claims us without our full knowledge or consent.

A number of challenges should continue to guide future research on the resignification of fatness. Fat scholars and activists persist in wrestling with the issue of designing actions and modes of representation that will indeed positively resignify the fat body, and in making contingency plans for the occasional backfire that turns their resignificatory efforts on their heads, leaving them further abjected. Theorizing about what might work, and why, and designing practical plans for dealing with the possible eventualities of risk are necessary steps in the project of reclaiming fat identity. We also must be dogged in our pursuit of an inhabitable subject position for fat people, always guarding against the easy slide back into subjection. This requires paying keen attention to the double-edged sword of resignificatory language games.

Though I and others have begun to get at some of these issues, much remains to be understood about the changing ways in which spoiled identities can be successfully resignified. Even if I were so bold as to declare a strategic answer to these challenges in light of what fat activists have accomplished, it would inevitably fall short of the job by the time the ink on this page had dried. In future research, what is most important is to continue to question our assumptions about the terms that discursively make or break bodies and to recognize that there is never a neat separation between the power we promote and that which we oppose.

Notes

Introduction

[1] I recognize the postwar era as an important time during which fat began to be understood as hugely problematic, while other scholars point to different periods during the twentieth century marked by cultural disdain for fat. Joan Jacobs Brumberg, for instance, contends that widespread contempt for fat came of age at the turn of the century, as newly "liberated" Victorians refocused their surveillance on their bodies instead of on their morals; see Brumberg, *The Body Project: An Intimate History of American Girls* (New York: Random House, 1997). I believe it is less important to pinpoint an exact moment for the beginning of fat hatred (an impossible task, anyhow) than it is to recognize the prevalence of this belief throughout the twentieth century, forcefully manifested at various key moments during the period.

Following Elizabeth Grosz, I want to be careful here *not* to suggest a lumpy body passively waiting to be signified by culture, for it is *through* culture that bodies are constructed. Although I feel that Grosz misrepresents the social constructionist project by equating it with the former, I am inclined to examine, as she recommends, how particular bodies are lived, "interwoven with and constitutive of systems of meaning, signification, and representation." Grosz, *Volatile Bodies: Toward a Corporeal Feminism* (Bloomington: Indiana University Press, 1994), 18.

[2] Melinda Beck, "An Epidemic of Obesity," *Newsweek*, (August 1, 1994), 63.

[3] Because I am working from a feminist framework, some might think it odd that I am not choosing to examine fat hatred as specifically anti-woman, given a historical (though viciously arbitrary) link between woman and the flesh. While it is the case that the vast majority of my research subjects identify as women, I want to be cautious about equating "fat" with "woman," as this connection is, at root, culturally constructed.

[4] Patricia Mann, *Micropolitics: Agency in a Postfeminist Era* (Minneapolis: University of Minnesota Press, 1994), 160.

[5] Paralleling Judith Butler's reading of Michel Foucault on sexed subjects, to say that fat subjects are innocent victims "is an illusory and complicitous conceit of emancipatory . . . politics." Butler, *Bodies That Matter: The Discursive Limits of "Sex"* (New York: Routledge, 1993), 97.

[6] Borrowing from John Stewart, interpersonal communication means something more than the common understanding of informal face-to-face communication between two or more people. Stewart defines interpersonal communication as "the quality of contact that occurs when the persons involved talk and listen in ways that maximize the presence of the personal." Stewart, *Bridges Not Walls: A Book about Interpersonal Communication*, 7th ed. (New York: McGraw-Hill, 1999), 15.

[7] Mann, *Micropolitics*, 22.

[8] Ibid., 31.

[9] Judith Butler, *Gender Trouble: Feminism and the Subversion of Identity* (New York: Routledge, 1990), 116.

[10] Ibid., 134.

[11] Ibid.

[12] Judith Butler, *Excitable Speech: A Politics of the Performative* (New York: Routledge, 1997), 5.

[13] This interest contrasts with the concern of many fat activists over finding *legal* remedies for the daily assaults on fat subjectivity. I am more interested in examining the cultural power of presentation and representation than in institutionalized legal or electoral power.

[14] Wittig, quoted in Butler, *Gender Trouble*, 115.

[15] Butler, *Gender Trouble*, 116.

[16] Ibid., 145.

[17] Butler, *Bodies That Matter*, 3.

[18] Grosz, *Volatile Bodies*, 19.

[19] Butler, *Bodies That Matter*, 21.

[20] Grosz, *Volatile Bodies*, 22.

[21] Ibid.

[22] Butler, *Gender Trouble*, 141.

[23] Ibid., 146–47.

[24] Grosz, *Volatile Bodies*, 19–20.

[25] The results of a recent Infotrac database search powered by the search term *fat* revealed only a few popular press articles (usually centered on dieting) and a bevy of journal selections on lipids. To find much of anything that deals with fat *bodies* rather than fat *molecules* in scholarly literature, one is required to search using the term *obesity*, already comfortably (but problematically) lodged in medical/scientific discourse.

[26] Grosz, *Volatile Bodies*, 35.

[27] Butler, *Gender Trouble*, viii–ix.

[28] Kristine L. Fitch, "Culture, Ideology, and Interpersonal Communication Research," in *Communication Yearbook* 17, ed. Stan A. Deetz (Thousand Oaks, Calif.: Sage, 1994), 107.

Chapter 1

[1] Though the temptation exists to focus specifically on *women's* fat bodies, and though most of my research subjects indeed identified themselves as women, I believe that the project of resignification of fatness is vital to (and is in part propelled by) men as well. Thus, my intentions are not gender specific.

[2] Mann, *Micropolitics*, 159.

[3] Eve Kosofsky Sedgwick and Michael Moon, "Divinity: A Dossier, a Performance Piece, a Little-Understood Emotion," in Eve Kosofsky Sedgwick, *Tendencies* (Durham, N.C.: Duke University Press, 1993).

[4] Elizabeth V. Spelman, *Inessential Woman: Problems of Exclusion in Feminist Thought* (Boston: Beacon, 1990), 58.

[5] Ibid., 60.

[6] Ibid., 62.

[7] Ibid., 113.

[8] Ibid., 68. Butler's take on the incompleteness of the term *women* is instructive: "If 'women' within political discourse can never fully describe that which it names, that is . . . because the term marks a dense intersection of social relations that cannot be summarized through the terms of identity." Butler, *Bodies That Matter*, 218.

9 Judith Butler, *Gender Trouble: Feminism and the Subversion of Identity* (New York: Routledge, 1990), 142.

10 Samuel R. Delany, "Street Talk/Straight Talk," *Differences: A Journal of Feminist Cultural Studies* 3, no. 2 (1991): 38.

11 Sarah Schulman, *My American History: Lesbian and Gay Life during the Reagan/Bush Years* (New York: Routledge, 1994), 279.

12 Gayle Rubin, "Thinking Sex: Notes for a Radical Theory of the Politics of Sexuality," in *Pleasure and Danger: Exploring Female Sexuality*, ed. Carole S. Vance (Boston: Routledge and Kegan Paul, 1984), 275.

13 Schulman, *My American History*, 279.

14 Eve Kosofsky Sedgwick, "Epistemology of the Closet," in *The Lesbian and Gay Studies Reader*, ed. Henry Abelove, Michèle Aina Barale, and David W. Halperin (New York: Routledge, 1993), 55.

15 Lisa Duggan, "Making It Perfectly Queer," *Socialist Review* 22, no. 1 (1992): 21–22, 20, 23.

16 Some might argue that while queer theory provides a kind of philosophical fuel for such play, it is queer *activists* who take action.

17 Exemplary of this last area are on-line sites and electronic mailing lists dedicated to fatness. On pro-fat Internet sites, users create narratives steeped in essentialist arguments and perspectives that suggest, instead, an understanding of their own subject position as the vortex constituted by a whirl of discourses.

18 Gloria Anzaldúa, *Borderlands/La Frontera: The New Mestiza* (San Francisco: Aunt Lute, 1987).

19 Cindy Patton, "Tremble Hetero Swine!," in *Fear of a Queer Planet: Queer Politics and Social Theory*, ed. Michael Warner (Minneapolis: University of Minnesota Press, 1993).

20 Butler, *Bodies That Matter*, 2.

21 For their focus on anorexic or bulimic women, see Joan Jacobs Brumberg, *Fasting Girls: The History of Anorexia Nervosa* (New York: Plume, 1989); Susie Orbach, *Hunger Strike* (London: Faber and Faber, 1986); and Carole Spitzack, *Confessing Excess: Women and the Politics of Body Reduction* (Albany: State University of New York Press, 1990). For imposition of food meanings, see Anne Scott Beller, *Fat and Thin: A Natural History of Obesity* (New York: Farrar, Straus and Giroux, 1977), and Naomi Wolf, *The Beauty Myth* (New York: Doubleday, 1991).

22 B. W. Thompson, " 'A Way Outa No Way': Eating Problems among African-American, Latina, and White Women," *Gender and Society* 6 (1992): 546–61.

23 For example, the work of the Fat Underground and the Lisa Schoenfielder/Barb Wieser anthology *Shadow on a Tightrope: Writings by Women on Fat Oppression* (San Francisco: Aunt Lute, 1983) sent small shock waves through a community whose primary feature of identification had been shame. Their work, along with that of the more moderate National Association to Advance Fat Acceptance (NAAFA), has helped in replacing this identity with a rhetoric of "fat rights."

24 I prefer to negotiate understanding through a grammar of artistic images and graphic representations rather than events or philosophies. In addition to its accessibility for the researcher, art is culturally and historically bound. Randall White maintains that "while we tend to think of art as evocative, that which is evoked depends heavily upon participation in a mutually understood system of meaning—in other words, a shared body of ideas, conceptions, and experiences. Far from being a universal language, art is culture-bound." Therefore, the negotiation of *images* presents a point of entry into understanding various historical and cultural conditions, as well as a challenge for the interpreter as "outsider." White, *Dark Caves, Bright Visions: Life in Ice Age Europe* (New York: Norton, 1986),

104. I originally selected these periods and regions for investigation because I believed that they hosted more appreciation for, or at least tolerance of, fatness than does most of North America at this point in time.

[25] Johannes Maringer and Hans-Georg Bandi, *Art in the Ice Age* (New York: Praeger, 1953), 28.

[26] Ibid., 28–29. Maringer's immediate labeling as "absurd" the possibility that a fat figure could invoke the name of Venus is a testament to the aesthetic narrowness of modernity. In an attempt to get beyond Maringer's socially constructed blinders, I choose to examine the possibility that fat was something valued positively in the Ice Age and was paid tribute to in representation.

[27] Ibid., 29.

[28] Laetitia LaFollette, personal communication; White, *Dark Caves*, 1986.

[29] Ibid., 127.

[30] Ibid.

[31] Arielle P. Kozloff and David Gordon Mitten, *The Gods Delight: The Human Figure in Classical Bronze* (Cleveland: Cleveland Museum of Art, 1988), 106.

[32] Ibid., 108. It is interesting here to compare Kozloff's refusal to consider Aphrodite as even slightly obese with the interpretation that would no doubt be rendered if Aphrodite were the object of the gaze of contemporary Americans; I suspect that the woman depicted in the sculpture would immediately be categorized as chubby—a rather less generous reading than Kozloff's "voluptuous," to be sure.

[33] Andrew Stewart, *Greek Sculpture: An Exploration,* 2 vols. (New Haven: Yale University Press, 1990), 1:79.

[34] Kozloff and Mitten, *The Gods Delight,* 154.

[35] Ibid., 158.

[36] Ibid., 115–16.

[37] Stewart, *Greek Sculpture,* 1:79.

[38] Ibid., 1:79, 78.

[39] Igor de Garine, preface to *Social Aspects of Obesity*, ed. Igor de Garine and Nancy J. Pollock (London: Gordon and Breach, 1995), x.

[40] Ibid.

[41] Victor Teti, "Food and Fatness in Calabria," in Garine and Pollock, *Social Aspects of Obesity*, 4, 25.

[42] See, respectively, Igor de Garine, "Sociocultural Aspects of the Male Fattening Sessions among the Massa of Northern Cameroon," P. J. Brink, "Fertility and Fat: The Annang Fattening Room," and Nancy J. Pollock, "Social Fattening Patterns in the Pacific: The Positive Side of Obesity—A Nauru Case Study," in Garine and Pollock, *Social Aspects of Obesity*.

[43] Garine, "Sociocultural Aspects."

[44] Brink, "Fertility and Fat," 83.

[45] Pollock, "Social Fattening Patterns," 88.

[46] Ibid., 93.

[47] Mary Douglas, *Purity and Danger* (New York: Praeger, 1966), 2.

[48] Ibid., 3.

[49] Ibid.

[50] It is noteworthy that Douglas does not consider the dangers of fluid exchanges between same-sex partners; perhaps this is a function of her pre-Stonewall 1966 publication date?

[51] Douglas, *Purity and Danger,* 4.

[52] Ibid.

⁵³ Ibid., 97.

⁵⁴ Ibid., 113.

⁵⁵ Victor Turner, *The Ritual Process* (Ithaca: Cornell University Press, 1977), following Arnold Van Gennep, *The Rites of Passage* (1909), trans. Monika B. Vizedom and Gabrielle L. Caffee (London: Routledge and Kegan Paul, 1960).

⁵⁶ This is one of those points at which fat-as-rite-of-passage slips a bit; does the fat subject "ambiguously slip through an interim cultural realm," or is the fat subject, more accurately, excluded? Turner's read on rites of passage is less suspicious, perhaps, than mine in this instance.

⁵⁷ Turner, *Ritual Process*, 95.

⁵⁸ Ibid.

⁵⁹ Ibid.

⁶⁰ Ibid., 97.

⁶¹ Sedgwick and Moon, "Divinity," 237.

Chapter 2

¹ Beck, "Epidemic of Obesity," 63.

² "Public Health: America's Getting Fatter," *American Journal of Nursing*, 94 no. 9 (1994): 9.

³ NIH Technology Assessment Conference Panel (hereafter NIH), "Methods for Voluntary Weight Loss and Control," *Annals of Internal Medicine* 119, no. 7 (October 1, 1993), p. 2: 764.

⁴ "Public Health," 9.

⁵ Ibid. It is important to note, though, that many fat activists dispute causal claims about obesity and diabetes, suggesting instead that metabolic irregularities in early-stage diabetes cause weight gain, rather than the reverse.

⁶ F. X. Pi-Sunyer, "Medical Hazards of Obesity," *Annals of Internal Medicine* 119, no. 7 (October 1, 1993), p. 2: 655.

⁷ Beck, "Epidemic of Obesity," 63.

⁸ Pi-Sunyer, "Medical Hazards of Obesity," 658.

⁹ NIH, "Methods," 770.

¹⁰ Ibid., 765.

¹¹ Ibid., 766, 768.

¹² Ibid.

¹³ William B. Carter, "Health Behavior as a Rational Process: Theory of Reasoned Action and Multiattribute Utility Theory," in *Health Behavior and Health Education: Theory, Research, and Practice*, ed. Karen Glanz, Frances M. Lewis, and Barbara K. Rimer (San Francisco: Jossey-Bass, 1990), 68.

¹⁴ Irwin M. Rosenstock, "The Health Belief Model: Explaining Health Behavior through Expectancies," in Glanz et al., *Health Behavior and Health Education*, 42–43.

¹⁵ N. Boucher, "Overfeds," *New Republic*, September 19, 1994, 36.

¹⁶ Ibid., 36.

¹⁷ Ornish, quoted in Beck, "Epidemic of Obesity," 63.

¹⁸ Boucher, "Overfeds," 36.

¹⁹ Ibid.

²⁰ NIH, "Methods," 767.

²¹ Ibid.

²² See R. W. Jeffery, "Minnesota Studies on Community-Based Approaches to Weight

Loss and Control," *Annals of Internal Medicine,* 119 no. 7 (October 1, 1993), p. 2: 719–21.

[23] Angela Kennedy, "Fair Deal? Fat Chance," *Nursing Standard* 9, no. 21 (February 15, 1995): 45.

[24] Carol T. Miller, Esther D. Rothblum, Diane Felicio, and Pamela Brand, "Compensating for Stigma: Obese and Nonobese Women's Reactions to Being Visible," *Personality and Social Psychology Bulletin* 21, no. 10 (October 1995): 1093. A recent happening exemplifying this "blame-the-fatty" mentality was the summer 2002 decision by Southwest Airlines to require fat passengers to pay two fares. For a satisfying take on the situation, see Lenore Skenazy, "Extra Fares for Fat Folk Are Flighty," *New York Daily News,* June 26, 2002, 33.

[25] NIH, "Methods," 764.

[26] Richard Klein, "Big Country," *New Republic,* September 19, 1994, 29.

[27] Ibid.

[28] See NIH, "Methods," 769.

[29] Klein, "Big Country," 32.

[30] Hanna Rosin, "Solid Citizens," *New Republic,* September 19, 1994, 26.

[31] Butler, *Gender Trouble,* 125; *NAAFA Newsletter,* December 1994/January 1995, 1.

[32] *NAAFA Newsletter,* December 1994/January 1995, 9.

[33] Ibid.

[34] Smith, in ibid.

[35] Lawrence Wallack, "Media Advocacy: Promoting Health through Mass Communication," in Glanz et al., *Health Behavior and Health Education,* 371.

[36] Ibid., 376. Social marketing is defined by Philip Kotler as "the design, implementation, and control of programs seeking to increase the acceptability of a social idea or practice in a target group." Kotler, *Marketing for Nonprofit Organizations* (Englewood Cliffs, N.J.: Prentice-Hall, 1982), 490.

[37] Wallack, "Media Advocacy," 377.

[38] Ibid., 378.

[39] Ibid., 379.

Chapter 3

[1] Of course, I concede that notions of "mainstream" and "alternative" are definitely fraught with difficulties; but for lack of something better, I use them. I should also make clear my methodological impulses during this examination of print media representations of fat, as it differs somewhat from the ethnographic perspective through which I analyzed the on-line data. After locating a relatively small number of representations of fat people which challenged traditional notions about their health, attractiveness, or sexuality, I engaged in textual analysis to present the interpretations in this section.

[2] Debbie Notkin, "Enlarging: Politics and Society," in Laurie Toby Edison and Debbie Notkin, *Women En Large: Images of Fat Nudes* (San Francisco: Books in Focus, 1994), 91.

[3] See Rosemary Bray, "Heavy Burden," *Essence,* January 1992, 53–54, 90–91; R. Brown, "Full-Figured Women Fight Back: Resistance Grows to Society's Demand for Slim Bodies," *Ebony,* March 1990, 27–31; and Vanessa Feltz, "Who Says Fat Isn't Sexy?," *Redbook,* December 1993, 45.

[4] Some critics characterize NAAFA as an organization with assimilationist tendencies, whereas the Fat Underground had more anarchic liberationist leanings. As I explain later, the assimilationist and the liberationist are not as far apart as they might at first seem; they both enable dominant structures to exist, in that the assimilationist tries to curry favor

within, while the liberationist tries to invert or transcend the structure. In later chapters, I examine the ways in which discursive resignifications of fatness work best—that is, when they imagine themselves to be retooling structures of health, nature, and beauty, rather than just fitting in with or escaping from them.

⁵ Bray, "Heavy Burden," 90.

⁶ Ibid., 90–91.

⁷ Roxanne Brown, "Full-Figured Women Fight Back," 28, 30.

⁸ Daniel Pinkwater, "I'm Going to Say It!," *Rump Parliament Magazine: Working to Change the Way Society Treats Fat People*, September 1994, 19.

⁹ Ibid.

¹⁰ This is not to ignore that the need to heal from very painful abuses takes priority over liberation; rather, it suggests that the very framing of fat existence as "abuse" dictates its reality as necessarily painful and negative.

¹¹ Vanessa Feltz, "Who Says Fat Isn't Sexy?," 45.

¹² Ibid.

¹³ Ibid.

¹⁴ Ibid.

¹⁵ Notkin, "Enlarging," 92.

¹⁶ Ibid., 97

¹⁷ Ibid., 98.

¹⁸ Alafonte, in ibid., 94. These goals, though, are flip sides of the same coin; as inseparable processes, it would seem that both need to happen for change to occur.

¹⁹ Susan Stinson, *Belly Songs: In Celebration of Fat Women* (Northampton, Mass.: Orogeny Press, 1993), 4–5.

²⁰ Ibid., 14–15, 16.

²¹ Ibid., 1.

²² FaT GiRL Publishing, *FaT GiRL: A Zine for Fat Dykes and the Women Who Want Them*, no. 1, 1994, 1.

²³ Mindy Ridgway, "Fat Dykes on Fat Dykes: Hot off the Press," *San Francisco Bay Times*, October 6, 1994, 7.

²⁴ *FaT GiRL*, no. 1, 13.

²⁵ Ibid., 14, 15.

²⁶ Ibid., 55.

²⁷ Michael Huspek, "Dueling Structures: The Theory of Resistance in Discourse," *Communication Theory* 3, no. 1 (1993): 2.

²⁸ Wendy Chapkis, *Beauty Secrets: Women and the Politics of Appearance* (Boston: South End Press, 1986), 14.

²⁹ Butler, *Gender Trouble*, 93.

³⁰ Chapkis, *Beauty Secrets*, 16.

³¹ Here, I mean that while the particular fashions of beauty are socially constructed and historically situated, the notion of *beauty itself* rarely gets questioned.

³² Chapkis, *Beauty Secrets*, 14.

³³ Susan Bordo, *Unbearable Weight: Feminism, Western Culture, and the Body* (Berkeley: University of California Press, 1993), 288.

³⁴ Ibid., 289.

³⁵ Ibid., 290.

³⁶ *FaT GiRL*, no. 1, 41.

³⁷ Bordo, *Unbearable Weight*, 292.

Chapter 4

[1] Hillel Schwartz, *Never Satisfied: A Cultural History of Diets, Fantasies, and Fat* (New York: Free Press, 1986), 4.

[2] Seymour Fisher, *Body Consciousness: You Are What You Feel* (Englewood Cliffs, N.J.: Prentice-Hall, 1973), 73.

[3] Chris Shilling, *The Body and Social Theory* (London: Sage, 1993), 41.

[4] For a fascinating and alarming report on attempts to alter the biological body in order to redress legal and material inequalities, see Craig S. Smith, "Risking Limbs for Height, and Success, in China," *New York Times*, May 5, 2002. Smith describes a surgery voluntarily undertaken by Chinese men and women desperate to be taller that requires intentionally broken bones and bed rest for extensive periods of time.

[5] Christian S. Crandall et al., "An Attribution-Value Model of Prejudice: Anti-Fat Attitudes in Six Nations," *Personality and Social Psychology Bulletin* 27, no. 1 (January 2001): 30–37. See also Diane M. Quinn and Jennifer Crocker, "When Ideology Hurts: Effects of Belief in the Protestant Ethic and Feeling Overweight on the Psychological Well-Being of Women," *Journal of Personality and Social Psychology* 77, no. 2 (August 1999): 402–14.

[6] Andrew Sullivan, "The Plump Classes Are on a Roll," *Sunday Times* (London), August 29, 1999.

[7] Mark Steyn, "Obestiality: America Has the Weight of Its Weight on Its Shoulders," *American Spectator* 31:56. Available at <http://www.spectator.org/archives/98-03_steyn .html>.

[8] See N. Allon, "The Stigma of Overweight in Everyday Life," in *Psychological Aspects of Obesity*, ed. B. B. Wolman (New York: Van Nostrand Reinhold, 1982), 130–74; also, G. Mann, "The Influence of Obesity on Health," *New England Journal of Medicine* 291 (1974): 178–85.

[9] Sander Gilman, *Picturing Health and Illness: Images of Identity and Difference* (Baltimore: Johns Hopkins University Press, 1995), 66.

[10] See Llewellyn Louderback, *Fat Power: Whatever You Weigh Is Right* (New York: Hawthorn, 1970), 25.

[11] Camryn Manheim, "If We're All a Little Pudgier in 2025, So What?," *Time*, November 8, 1999, 90.

[12] Schwartz, *Never Satisfied*, 329.

[13] G. Searle, *The Quest for National Efficiency* (Oxford: Basil Blackwell, 1971), cited in Shilling, *Body and Social Theory*, 30.

[14] Schwartz, *Never Satisfied*, 142.

[15] Leslie D. Haravon, "Gaining Respect: Fat Women and Resistance," (Ph.D. diss., University of Iowa, 1996), 45.

[16] Nomy Lamm, "Fishnets, Feather Boas, and Fat," in *Adiós, Barbie: Young Women Write about Body Image and Identity*, ed. Ophira Edut (Seattle: Seal Press, 1998), 80. Lamm was one of *Ms.* magazine's Women of the Year in 1997.

[17] Mary Russo, *The Female Grotesque: Risk, Excess, and Modernity* (London: Routledge, 1995), 23.

[18] Elizabeth Birmingham, "Fearing the Freak: How Talk TV Articulates Women and Class," *Journal of Popular Film and Television* 28, no. 3 (Fall 2000): 133+.

[19] Jonathan Wise and Susan Kierr Wise, *The Overeaters: Eating Styles and Personality* (New York: Human Sciences Press, 1979), 140.

[20] Medina et al. argue that Mexican Americans are less able to delay gratification (in terms of consumer spending behavior) than Anglo-Americans. Dinesh D'Souza claims that poor blacks have contempt for deferred gratification, and Michael Sigfried maintains that

American inner cities are in shambles partly because of the focus on the immediate present held by their residents, whom one infers to be minority group members. See José F. Medina, Joel Saegert, and Alicia Gresham, "Comparison of Mexican-American and Anglo-American Attitudes toward Money," *Journal of Consumer Affairs* 30 (Summer 1996): 124–45; Dinesh D'Souza, "The National Prospect," *Commentary,* November 1995, 47–48; and Michael L. Siegfried, "The Inner City in the 21ˢᵗ Century: Huxley's Brave New World Revisited," *Journal of Interdisciplinary Studies* 8, nos. 1–2 (1996): 19–30.

[21] Wise and Wise, *Overeaters,* 202.

[22] Jane Ogden concurs: "It is necessary for the dieting industry to sell the idea that fat means a problem so that they can go about solving this problem. However, it is a problem that they themselves have created." Ogden, *Fat Chance! The Myth of Dieting Explained* (London: Routledge, 1992), 12.

[23] Pierre Bordieu, "The Forms of Capital," in *Handbook of Theory and Research for the Sociology of Education,* ed. J. Richardson (New York: Greenwood Press, 1986), cited in Shilling, *Body and Social Theory,* 133.

[24] Pierre Bordieu, *Distinction: A Social Critique of the Judgment of Taste,* trans. Richard Nice (Cambridge: Harvard University Press, 1987), 193.

[25] Shilling, *Body and Social Theory,* 139.

[26] Leslie A. Fiedler, "The Tyranny of the Normal," in *The Tyranny of the Normal: An Anthology,* ed. Carol Donley and Sheryl Buckley (Kent, Ohio: Kent State University Press, 1996), 10.

[27] Louderback, *Fat Power,* 79.

[28] D. Kinder and D. O. Sears, "Prejudice and Politics: Symbolic Racism versus Racial Threats to the Good Life," *Journal of Personality and Social Psychology* 40 (1981): 414–31, cited in Christian S. Crandall, "Prejudice Against Fat People: Ideology and Self Interest," *Journal of Personality and Social Psychology* 66, (1994): 888.

[29] Cited in Natalie Angier, "Who Is Fat? It Depends on Culture: Culture and Status," *New York Times,* November 7, 2000, F1.

[30] The study was carried out by the New England Regional Genetics Group; cited in Janet Weeks, "Activists Plan a 'No-Diet Day,' " *St. Louis Post Dispatch,* May 2, 1994, 4D.

[31] Donna Allegra, "Fat Dancer," in *Journeys to Self Acceptance: Fat Women Speak,* ed. Carol Wiley (Freedom, Calif.: Crossing Press, 1994), 109.

[32] Cited in Mimi Nichter, *Fat Talk: What Girls and Their Parents Say about Dieting* (Cambridge,: Harvard University Press, 2000), 159. See, for example, K. S. Kemper, R. G. Sargent, J. W. Drane, R. F. Valois, and J. R. Hussey, "Black and White Females' Perceptions of Ideal Body Size and Social Norms," *Obesity Research* 2 (1994): 117–26 and M. Story, S. French, M. Resnick, and R. Blum, "Ethnic/Racial and Socioeconomic Differences in Dieting Behaviors and Body Image Perceptions in Adolescents," *International Journal of Eating Disorders* 18, no. 2 (1995): 173–79.

[33] Nichter, *Fat Talk,* 163.

[34] Ibid., 167–68. See also Joan E. Dolamore, "Living Large: The Experiences of Black and White Women of Being Fat in the United States" (Ph.D. diss., Harvard University, 1999), who contends that instead of small body size, commitment to her community is the marker of a black woman's worth.

[35] Henri E. Cauvin, "South Africa Confronts Another Health Problem: Obesity," *New York Times,* December 19, 2000, F1.

[36] Ibid.

[37] Cited in Marisa Urgo for the Office of Minority Health—U.S. Department of Health and Human Services, "Closing the Gap," 1998, 6.

[38] T. J. Bryan, "The Perfect Fit?," *Fireweed* 67, Fat Issue, (1999): 38–45, 43.

[39] Schwartz, *Never Satisfied*, 330.

[40] Regina D. Williams, "Conquering the Fear of a Fat Body: The Journey toward Myself," in *Adiós, Barbie: Young Women Write about Body Image and Identity*, ed. Ophira Edut (Seattle: Seal Press, 1998), 178.

[41] See Anne C. Beal, "Weighty Matters," *Essence*, January 2001, 123–24.

[42] Ibid., 124.

[43] See ibid. Also see M. B. Harris, L. C. Walters, and S. Waschull, "Gender and Ethnic Differences in Obesity-Related Behaviors and Attitudes in a College Sample," *Journal of Applied Social Psychology* 21 (1991): 1545–77; Ophira Edut and Negar Mahmoodzadegan, "The Big Picture: Do Black Women Have Better Body Image Than White Women?," *Hues*, January 31, 1996, 39; and C. E. Rucker III and T. F. Cash, "Body Images, Body Size Perceptions, and Eating Behavior among African-Americans and White College Women," *International Journal of Eating Disorders* 12 (1992): 291–99. Note that a recent study indicates that African American women are no more satisfied with their body sizes than are Caucasian women and that African American men are no different from Caucasian men in the female shapes that they find most attractive. See Jack Demarest, "Body Image: Gender, Ethnic, and Age Differences," *Journal of Social Psychology* 140, no. 4 (August 2000): 465+.

[44] Elisa J. Sobo, "The Sweetness of Fat: Health, Procreation, and Sociability in Rural Jamaica," in *Many Mirrors: Body Image and Social Relations*, ed. Nicole Sault (New Brunswick, N.J.: Rutgers University Press, 1994), 139.

[45] Charlotte Cooper, *Fat and Proud: The Politics of Size* (London: Women's Press, 1998), 43.

[46] Shilling, *Body and Social Theory*, 5.

[47] Schwartz, *Never Satisfied*, 325.

[48] Cooper, *Fat and Proud*, 6.

[49] Martinez-Regino, quoted in Lisa Belkin, "Watching Her Weight," *New York Times Magazine*, July 8, 2001, 32.

[50] Affidavit, quoted in ibid.

[51] Pritchard, quoted in ibid., 33.

Chapter 5

[1] This text is taken from the back of a postcard featuring Ruby (the aforementioned doll) which I bought at the Body Shop, 1997.

[2] For an account of Manheim's Emmy experience and her battles with fat oppression, see Paul Brownfield, "She's Made Her Case a Bit Too Well: Camryn Manheim Has Found Fame as a Lawyer on 'The Practice' and as a Challenger of the 'Thin Is In' Credo," *Los Angeles Times*, June 20, 1999, 8.

[3] Danae Clark, "Commodity Lesbianism," *Camera Obscura* 25 (January 1991): 179–201.

[4] Goldblatt et al., quoted in Wise and Wise, *Overeaters*, 155. I use the author's term *obese* in this context, though I find it objectionable as an artifact of anti-fat medical discourse. Noteworthy in her opposition to arguments about why poor people tend to be fat is Charlotte Cooper, who rejects such studies because they suggest an inappropriate relationship to food and a sense that fat people are responsible for their body size. See Cooper, *Fat and Proud*.

[5] Marcela Valente, "Rights-Argentina: Legislating Larger Clothing Sizes for Women," *Interpress Service*, March 8, 2000.

[6] The Forgotten Woman is now an upscale boutique chain catering to fat women.

[7] Chris Hansen, Lane Bryant marketing executive, quoted in Courtney Kane, "A Male Sex Symbol Enjoys the Company of Larger Women in a New Campaign for Lane Bryant," *New York Times*, February 1, 2001, C8. Also see "ShopKo's Plus-Plus (Size) Situation," *DSN Retailing Today* 39, no. 18 (September 18, 2000): A8–A10.

[8] Quoted in Suzanne S. Brown, "It's Fitting: Fashion Embraces Full-Sized Women," *Denver Post*, November 2, 2000, A20.

[9] Pactor, quoted in ibid.

[10] LeWinter, quoted in Erika D. Peterman, "A Big Idea Catches On: Trendy Clothes in Plus Sizes," *Los Angeles Times*, November 19, 1999, 1.

[11] Valente, "Rights-Argentina." But before you get too excited, note Valente's report that parliamentary deputy Maria del Carmen Banzas explains "that the law was designed to get manufacturers 'to offer all normal anthropometric sizes, not extra-large sizes for obese people.' "

[12] Girlfriends LA catalog, Spring 2001. Available from <www.gfla.com>.

[13] Abigail Goldman, "Chain Sees Big Business in Larger Sizes: Lane Bryant Has Been Remaking Its Image to Capture More of the Market Catering to 'Realistic Body Sizes,' " *Los Angeles Times*, June 25, 1999, 1.

[14] Hansen, quoted in Kane, "A Male Sex Symbol," 18.

[15] This resembles the taming of female bodybuilders described by Laurie Schulze, as summarized by Clark, "Commodity Lesbianism," 195.

[16] Ibid.

[17] Quoted in Ophira Edut, "Filling Out Fashion—The Expanding Plus-Size Fashion Scene," *Hues*, December 31, 1998, 18.

[18] Cooper, *Fat and Proud*, 157–58.

[19] Haravon, "Gaining Respect," 121.

[20] Nomy Lamm, "I Love Dressing Up," *Ms.*, April/May 1999, 12.

[21] See Edut, "Filling Out Fashion."

[22] Mariko Tamaki, "Angry Naked Fat Woman," *Fireweed* 67, Fat Issue (1999): 25.

[23] Ibid., 26.

[24] Flaque, quoted in Marilyn Wann, "Women: Self-Hatred and Celery Sticks. Life Is Too Short for Either," *Guardian* (Manchester), March 29, 1999, T007.

[25] Wann, "Women: Self-Hatred and Celery Sticks."

[26] Prices and items are quoted in Linda Gillan Griffin, "Plus Sizes, Plus Style, Plus Profits," *Houston Chronicle*, January 18, 2000, 1: For pay penalty statistic, see Gina Kolata, "The Burdens of Being Overweight: Mistreatment and Misconceptions," *New York Times*, November 22, 1992, A1.

[27] Edut, "Filling Out Fashion."

[28] Nita McKinley, "Ideal Weight/Ideal Women: Society Constructs the Female," in *Weighty Issues: Fatness and Thinness as Social Problems*, ed. Jeffery Sobal and Donna Maurer (New York: Aldine de Gruyter, 1999), 111.

[29] I echo Clark's treatment of the plight of lesbian consumers in "Commodity Lesbianism," 192.

[30] Ehrenstein, quoted in Clark, "Commodity Lesbianism," 192.

[31] Erin Keating, "What's the Big Deal? Erin Keating Reflects on the Bold 'n' Fleshy Frontier of *Mode* Magazine," *Bitch: Feminist Response to Pop Culture*, 3 no. 2 (July 1998): 34.

[32] Clark, "Commodity Lesbianism," 192.

[33] Ophira Edut points out the problem here: "Since the majority of U.S. women are plus-size, are we really just repackaging 'average' women into a new consumer order? We're marketing products to the masses—a sound business decision, but hardly a subversive political act." "Filling Out Fashion."

[34] Goldman, "Chain Sees Big Business."

[35] Such shrinking parallels developments on the "regular" size (ha!) runway; Meghan Cox Gurdon reports that in 1998 "Chanel model Karen Elson (32-24-34) was dropped from Dolce & Gabbana's Milan runway because she was thought 'too fat' for the clothes." Gurdon, "The Real Skinny on Why We Feel Fat," *Women's Quarterly,* Summer 2000.

[36] Alex Kuczynksi, "The Incredible Shrinking Plus-Size Model," *New York Times,* March 29, 1998, sec. 9, 4.

[37] Edut, "Filling Out Fashion."

[38] Keating, "What's the Big Deal?"

[39] Dr. Thomas Szasz, *The Manufacture of Madness,* cited in Llewellyn Louderback, *Fat Power: Whatever You Weigh Is Right* (New York: Hawthorn, 1970), 203.

[40] Clark, "Commodity Lesbianism," 193.

[41] Here, Shilling (*Body and Social Theory,* 143), draws on the work of Mike Featherstone. See Featherstone, "Perspectives on Consumer Culture," *Sociology* 24, no. 1 (1990): 5–22.

Chapter 6

[1] Rosemarie Garland-Thomson, *Extraordinary Bodies: Figuring Physical Disability in American Culture and Literature* (New York: Columbia University Press, 1997), 6.

[2] Michael Bérubé, "Foreword: Pressing the Claim," in Simi Linton, *Claiming Disability: Knowledge and Identity* (New York: New York University Press, 1998), vii.

[3] Susan Peters, "The Politics of Disability Identity," in *Disability and Society: Emerging Issues and Insights,* ed. Len Barton (New York: Addison Wesley Longman, 1996), 216.

[4] Garland-Thomson, *Extraordinary Bodies,* 7.

[5] Paul Darke, "Understanding Cinematic Representations of Disability," in *The Disability Reader: Social Science Perspectives,* ed. Tom Shakespeare (London: Cassell, 1998), 182.

[6] Ibid., 183.

[7] Ibid., 190.

[8] Chris Hicks, "Movie Review: What's Eating Gilbert Grape," on Deseret News website, <http://deseretnews.com/movies/view/1,1257,1994,00.html>. Reviewed on March 4, 1994; retrieved on October 27, 2000.

[9] Simi Linton, *Claiming Disability: Knowledge and Identity* (New York: New York University Press, 1998), 3.

[10] J. R. Hanks and L. M. Hanks Jr., "The Physically Handicapped in Certain Non-Occidental Societies," *Journal of Social Issues* 13 (1948): 11–20, reworked in Linton, ibid., 38.

[11] Linton, *Claiming Disability,* 112.

[12] Ibid., 38.

[13] Jerome E. Bickenbach, *Physical Disability and Social Policy* (Toronto: University of Toronto Press, 1993), 71, cited in Jane Campbell and Mike Oliver, *Disability Politics: Understanding Our Past, Changing Our Future* (New York: Routledge, 1996), 179.

Chapter 7

[1] Cooper, *Fat and Proud,* 82.

[2] Michelle Joy Levine, *I Wish I Were Thin, I Wish I Were Fat* (New York: Fireside Books, 1999).

[3] Robert Pool, *FAT: Fighting the Obesity Epidemic* (New York: Oxford, 2001), 14.

[4] Barbara McFarland and Tyeis Baker-Baumann, "Shame and Body Image: Culture

and the Compulsive Eater," in *The Tyranny of the Normal: An Anthology,* ed. Carol Donley and Sheryl Buckley (Kent, Ohio: Kent State University Press, 1996), 107. For a different perspective—that it is only the minority of fat people who overeat to reduce sexual-social tensions—see Colleen S. W. Rand, "Obesity and Human Sexuality," *Medical Aspects of Human Sexuality* 13, no. 1 (1979): 141–52. Another classic study found no difference in the sexual functioning of fat and thin women, other than that fat women had a slightly higher percentage of orgasms. See A. H. Crisp, "The Possible Significance of Some Behavioral Correlates of Weight and Carbohydrate Intake," *Journal of Psychosomatic Research* 11, no. 117 (1967).

⁵ Amy Kaiser, "Safety in Pounds," *Moxie,* Summer 1999.

⁶ Barry D. Adam, *The Survival of Domination* (New York: Elsevier North Holland, 1978), cited in Edwin M. Schur, *The Politics of Deviance: Stigma Contests and the Uses of Power* (Englewood Cliffs, N.J.: Prentice-Hall, 1980), 146.

⁷ Alex Comfort, ed., *The Joy of Sex: A Gourmet Guide to Love Making* (New York: Fireside Books, 1972), 246.

⁸ McKinley, "Ideal Weight/Ideal Women," 105.

⁹ Gilman, *Picturing Health and Illness,* 62.

¹⁰ Catherine Manton, *Fed Up: Women and Food in America* (Westport, Conn.: Bergin and Garvey, 1999), 91. See also Annie Fursland, "Eve Was Framed: Food and Sex and Women's Shame," in *Fed Up and Hungry: Women, Oppression, and Food,* ed. Marilyn Lawrence (New York: Peter Bedrick Books, 1987), 23.

¹¹ Alexander Doty, "The Sissy Boy, the Fat Ladies, and the Dykes: Queerness and/as Gender in Pee-wee's World," *Camera Obscura* 25 (January 1991): 130.

¹² Beller cites an unpublished study done by William Shipman and L. Schwartz of Michael Reese Hospital in Chicago; see Beller, *Fat and Thin,* 74–75.

¹³ Ibid., 78.

¹⁴ Celia McCrea and Maurice Yaffe, "Sexuality in the Obese," *British Journal of Sexual Medicine* 8, no. 69 (February 1981): 37.

¹⁵ Hanne Blank, *Big Big Love: A Sourcebook on Sex for People of Size and Those Who Love Them,* (Emeryville, Calif.: Greenery Press, 2000), 64.

¹⁶ Ibid., 11.

¹⁷ Schur, *The Politics of Deviance,* 151. Llewellyn Louderback also warns fat people about letting their fat overwhelm all other aspects of their personality: "Like certain homosexuals, they become caricatures of themselves. They stress their differences, their weaknesses." Louderback, *Fat Power,* 197.

¹⁸ Patrick Giles, "A Matter of Size," in *Looking Queer: Body Image and Identity in Lesbian, Bisexual, Gay, and Transgender Communities,* ed. Dawn Atkins (Binghamton, N.Y.: Haworth, 1998), 355–56.

¹⁹ Ganapati S. Durgadas, "Fatness and the Feminized Man," in Atkins, *Looking Queer,* 368.

²⁰ Ibid., 370.

²¹ Witness, for example, the following personals from the "Women Seeking Women" section of the *Village Voice* on-line: "Attractive 30ish African American attr female seeking attractive femme F who is looking for a serious relationship. D/D free. No dykes or heavies please. Must be serious minded. No baggage please." Another advertiser specifies her preferences using slightly more coded wording: "Attractive Italian, 39, 5'5" 138lbs with an interest in having her first bi experience ISO attractive, slim white Female 30–40 yrs old. D&D free." *Village Voice* personals, available at <http://www.villagevoice.com/personals/>, posted August 7, 2001; retrieved August 8, 2001.

²² Alex Robertson Textor, "Organization, Specialization, and Desires in the Big Men's

Movement: Preliminary Research in the Study of Subculture-Formation," *Journal of Gay, Lesbian, and Bisexual Identity* 4, no. 3 (July 1999): 234.

²³ Tan, quoted in Blank, *Big Big Love*, 54.

²⁴ Andrew J. Feraios, "If Only I Were Cute: Looksism and Internalized Homophobia in the Gay Male Community," in Atkins, *Looking Queer*, 429.

²⁵ Textor, "Organization, Specialization," 219.

²⁶ An interesting discussion of fat men's preference for the moniker of "big men" within the Girth and Mirth context can be found in Jim Merrett, "The Size of the Matter: After Years of Being Settled for, Big Men Come into Their Own," *Advocate*, October 22, 1991, 60–61: "While not particularly political, big men's clubs are militant about one thing: Their members don't like to be called fat. 'No matter what anybody says,' notes Ronald Savaria . . . 'the word *fat* is offensive. We aren't fat, we're big.' Although a few radicals are working to rehabilitate the word *fat* the way other gays have co-opted *queer*, the majority of Girth and Mirth members prefer to be called big or heavy men, chubby, chubette, and superchub."

²⁷ Van Lynn Floyd in the January/February 1994 issue of *Bulk Male*, as cited in Textor, "Organization, Specialization," 223.

²⁸ Les Wright, *The Bear Book: Readings in the History and Evolution of a Gay Male Subculture* (New York: Haworth, 1997), 22.

²⁹ John Peebles in the September/October 1994 issue of *Bulk Male*, as cited in Textor, "Organization, Specialization," 224.

³⁰ Ray Kampf, *The Bear Handbook: A Comprehensive Guide for Those Who Are Husky, Hairy, and Homosexual and Those Who Love 'Em* (New York: Harrington Park, 2000), 44.

³¹ Wright, *Bear Book*, 34.

³² Textor, "Organization, Specialization," 226.

³³ Ibid., 227.

³⁴ Blank, *Big Big Love*, 240–42. Note, though, that disgust for feederism (an erotic practice involving feeders, who are aroused by observing eating and weight gain, and feedees, who are aroused by eating, being fed, and gaining weight) is overwhelming compared with suspicion of fat admirers, because of the frequently predatory nature of feeders in acquiring feedees. For an example of publicly expressed feminist disgust with feederism, see Camryn Manheim, *Wake Up! I'm Fat!* (New York: Broadway Books, 1999): "It really devastates me that there are women who are so lonely and so sad that they will allow and invite this kind of abuse. And it really pisses me off that there are men who are willing to take advantage of this loneliness to act out their fantasies of domination and dehumanization"(131–33).

³⁵ For more on this phenomenon, see Erich Goode and Joanne Preissler, "Admirers of Fat Women," *Medical Aspects of Human Sexuality* 16, no. 3 (1982): 140–45.

³⁶ Nichter, *Fat Talk*, 47.

³⁷ See Warren Johansson and William A. Percy, *Outing: Shattering the Conspiracy of Silence* (New York: Haworth, 1994), for an extensive treatment of the cases for and against outing.

³⁸ Brownfield, "She's Made Her Case," 8.

³⁹ Ibid.

⁴⁰ In a private interview, Jones says, "I've never had issues surrounding my size. It's only since I've been on 'The View' that peole seem more concerned about the size of my butt than the size of my brain." Sylvia Rubin, " 'The View's' Star Jones Shares Her Fashion Savvy," *San Francisco Chronicle*, May 9, 2000, E6. See also "Large and in Charge: Full-Figured Celebrities Proud of Their Stature," *Jet*, April 17, 2000, 52–57.

⁴¹ "Large and in Charge," 53.

[42] Beth Bernstein and Matilda St. John, "The Roseanne Benedict Arnolds," *Bitch: Feminist Response to Pop Culture*, no. 13 (2001): 43–47, 106–07.

[43] Disturbingly, Carnie Wilson's star power seems to have increased because of her gastric bypass and ensuing plastic surgery—not because of any recent singing on her part. For sycophantic reporting on Wilson, see the cover story by Sophfronia Scott and Ulrica Wihlborg, "Finishing Touches," *People Weekly*, June 17, 2002, 96–102.

[44] Bernstein and St. John, "Roseanne Benedict Arnolds," 106.

[45] Amy Walton, "Fat Girl Walking," *Fireweed* 67, Fat Issue (1999): 57.

[46] Pam Hinden, "The Fats of Life: Reflections on the Tyranny of Fatophobia," *Off Our Backs: A Women's Newsjournal*, March 31, 1983, 30.

[47] Cooper, *Fat and Proud*, 44.

[48] Ibid., 144.

[49] Marilyn Wann, in Oliver Burkeman, "We're Here and We're Spheres!," *Guardian* (Manchester), August 25, 1998, 7.

[50] Quoted in Greg Winter, "Fraudulent Marketers Capitalize on Demand for Sweat-Free Diets," *New York Times*, October 29, 2000, see 1, 1.

[51] Extracted from Lamm's zine, cited in Roxy Walker, "The Next Generation of Activists: Frank, Thoughtful, Articulate," *Radiance: The Magazine for Large Women*, Summer 1995, 8.

[52] Thanks to Julie Tokash for locating Lake's commentary on her icon status. See <www.brassring.com>.

[53] Leanne Cusitar et al. "Big Fat Editorial," *Fireweed* 67, Fat Issue (Fall 1999): 6–7.

[54] Mary Willmuth argues that despite evidence that fat people are no more psychologically disturbed than average-weight people, their experiences of discrimination, humiliation, and isolation may contribute to depression and even paranoia. Willmuth, "Treatment of Obesity: A Socio-Political Perspective," *Women and Therapy* 5, no. 4 (December 31, 1986): 27.

[55] Lamm, "Fishnets, Feather Boas, and Fat," 82.

Chapter 8

[1] Butler, *Gender Trouble*, 132.

[2] According to Judith Butler, "the abject designates those 'unlivable' and 'uninhabitable' zones of social life which are nevertheless densely populated by those who do not enjoy the status of the subject, but whose living under the sign of the 'unlivable' is required to circumscribe the domain of the subject." Butler, *Bodies That Matter*, 3.

[3] Mann, *Micropolitics*, 27.

[4] Nancy Fraser, "Rethinking the Public Sphere: A Contribution to the Critique of Actually Existing Democracy," in *Habermas and the Public Sphere*, ed. Craig Calhoun (Cambridge: MIT Press, 1992), 109–142.

[5] I use the abbreviations *FAS* and *FD* instead of the full names of the newsgroup and the list. Though privacy was not mentioned as a huge concern for those on the public *FAS* bulletin board, many members of *FD* expressed concern about the maintenance of their privacy on what was considered by some to be their "private" electronic mailing list. Thus, I agreed to conceal the name of the group.

[6] NIH, "Methods for Voluntary," 765. This phenomenon is not limited to adults; popular sources in recent years have reported as many as 80 percent of fourth-grade schoolgirls as engaging in dieting behavior.

[7] One *FAS* subscriber portrays the list as composed of classic overachievers: "I've heard of an inordinate number of graduate degrees on this board (I'm working on my third right now). I also posted a few weeks ago that I had noticed that whenever I come into work on a holiday or weekend, or early or late, it is the larger people who are here, never the thin

ones. . . . And it isn't because we don't have lives outside of work. . . .It seems that the only thing we forego is sleep." *FAS*, June 26, 1996. One might also make an educated guess that the participants benefit from some degree of social class advantage, given their knowledge of computer use and their relative ease of access to computer equipment.

[8] Of course, one could argue that if *no one* took responsibility for starting new threads and responding to others, the groups would disintegrate; however, this has not been a salient issue. Still, there are times when technical glitches have caused posts to "disappear," thus prompting disappointed members to complain about a lack of response, which is usually quickly remedied by simply resending the message(s).

[9] The word *fit* here is able to be plumbed both for literal and metaphorical meaning: fat people are often criticized for their physical inability to fit within the "proper" dimensions of a human body. Intolerance of this lack of fit creates stigma, thus making the fat person ill-fitted for social relationships as well.

[10] *FD*, April 14, 1997.

[11] *FD*, April 20, 1997; *FD*, June 21, 1996.

[12] *FD*, September 11, 1995.

[13] *FD*, June 19, 1996.

[14] *FAS*, April 24, 1997.

[15] *FD*, March 6, 1997.

[16] *FD*, April 15, 1997.

[17] *FD*, July 19, 1996.

[18] *FD*, April 16, 1997.

[19] *FD*, April 16, 1997.

[20] *FD*, February 10, 1998.

[21] One *FD* member says that "when average sized women say they are fat, it makes above average sized women mad. There is no universally agreed on weight that divides the average sized from the fat, and fat includes a very wide range of sizes. The same average sized woman who calls herself too fat will rush to tell you you are not fat if you make a good appearance and she likes you" (*FD*, February 5, 1998).

[22] *FD*, April 2, 1996.

[23] *FD*, March 7, 1997.

[24] *FD*, April 18, 1997.

[25] Schulman, *My American History*.

[26] One *FAS* post recommended Kaz Cooke's book *Real Gorgeous*, which prescribes sending the following type of letter to fashion magazine editors: "Dear Editor, the model on page 72 of your latest issue looks like a sick whippet. I want to know what the clothes look like on a size 14. And PS, please give that model some lunch before she faints. Signed, Reasonably Outraged, Come to Think About It." *FAS*, March 8, 1997.

[27] *FD*, March 6, 1997.

[28] *FD*, February 8, 1998.

[29] Elizabeth Grosz, *Space, Time, and Perversion: Essays on the Politics of Bodies* (New York: Routledge, 1995), 62.

[30] Mann, *Micropolitics*, 158.

[31] Butler, *Gender Trouble*, x.

[32] Ibid., 223.

[33] William Safire explains the origins of "phat": "Though some have postulated the origin of *phat* as an acronym for 'pretty hips and thighs' or even more lascivious constructions, the word is more likely a deliberate misspelling of *fat*, which has for centuries had a slang meaning of 'rich,' as in 'fat and happy.' " "All Phat! and a Bag of Chips," *New York Times Magazine*, May 17, 1998, 30.

[34] Butler, *Gender Trouble*, 124.

[35] Ibid., 127.

[36] Butler, *Bodies That Matter*, 193.

[37] Ibid., 219.

[38] Ibid., 221–22.

Chapter 9

[1] See <www.yourmom.com>, accessed January 18, 2001.

[2] Steyn, "Obestiality," 54.

[3] Jane G. Bacon and Beatrice E. Robinson, "Fat Phobia and the F-Scale—Measuring, Understanding, and Changing Anti-Fat Attitudes," *Melpomene Journal* 16, no. 1 (Spring 1997): 24+.

[4] Studies cited in Foster Klug, "Triathlete Won't Let Fat Get in the Way of Fit," *Los Angeles Times*, January 28, 2001, B4.

[5] Steven Blair, quoted in Klug, "Triathlete," B4.

[6] Gina Kolata, "While Children Grow Fatter, Experts Search for Solutions: Learning to Eat," *New York Times*, October 19, 2000, A1.

[7] Natalie Angier, "Who Is Fat? It Depends on Culture: Culture and Status," *New York Times*, November 7, 2000, F1.

[8] Ibid.

[9] Ibid.

[10] See studies cited in Jane Ogden, *Fat Chance! The Myth of Dieting Explained* (London: Routledge, 1992), 8. For a more personal explanation of the "I eat moderately, exercise strenuously, and am still fat" variety, see Ruth Raymond Thone, *Fat—A Fate Worse Than Death? Women, Weight and Appearance* (New York: Haworth, 1997).

[11] Sondra Solovay, *Tipping the Scales of Justice: Fighting Weight-Based Discrimination* (Amherst, N.Y.: Prometheus, 2000).

[12] Ibid., 19.

[13] Ibid., 195.

[14] Haravon, "Gaining Respect," 105–06.

[15] Attributed to Dr. Katherine Flegal in Kolata, "While Children Grow," A1.

[16] Solovay, *Tipping the Scales*, 153–54. See also Wendy Chapkis, "Freaks, Fairies, and Fat Ladies: A Right to Discriminate?," *Critical Sociology* 20, no. 3 (1994): 148–54.

[17] A happy exception to this comes in the case of Jennifer Portnick, a 240-pound aerobics instructor who sued Jazzercise after being rejected as an employee because of her size. Portnick won as a result of her argument that her skills were never questioned, just her size. See Patricia Leigh Brown, "240 Pounds, Persistent and Jazzercise's Equal," *New York Times*, May 8, 2002, A20. For a legal perspective on the general issue, see Michelle A. Travis, "Perceived Disabilities, Social Cognition, and 'Innocent Mistakes,' " *Vanderbilt Law Review*, March 2002, 55 Vand. L. Rev 481. Available via LexisNexis.

[18] Solovay, *Tipping the Scales*, 190.

[19] Butler, *Excitable Speech*, and Donna Haraway, "A Manifesto for Cyborgs: Science, Technology, and Socialist Feminism in the 1980s," in *Feminism/Postmodernism*, ed. Linda Nicholson (New York: Routledge, 1990).

[20] Chapkis, "Freaks, Fairies, and Fat Ladies," 153.

[21] Marilyn Wann, *Fat! So? Because You Don't Have to Apologize for Your Size!* (Berkeley, Calif: Ten Speed Press, 1998), 84.

[22] Bryan, "Perfect Fit?," 38–45, 44.

[23] Cooper, *Fat and Proud*, 43. This sentiment is echoed by Bovey, who says, "I do not

believe Big is Beautiful. I believe it is normal and therefore worthy of the same unexceptional treatment as those whom society already considers normal. I would like to see fat people accorded a validity which has nothing to do with their size or their looks." *The Forbidden Body: Why Being Fat Is Not a Sin* (London: Pandora, 1994), 189.

[24] Russo, *Female Grotesque*, 76.

[25] *FD*, July 20, 1996.

[26] *FD*, July 21, 1996.

[27] *FD*, July 21, 1997.

[28] Ibid. A response to this idea of "butt-saving" that I quite liked: "I think that's just fine, because coming out in any way you want to do it is a brave act, and can certainly have dire repercussions, and I also will certainly protect my ass whenever possible. . . . I am nothing if not situational in my ethics. . . . I'm capable of full-blown action-adventure LIES if the situation calls for it." *FD*, July 22, 1996.

[29] Here, I am paralleling a concern over Sharon Marcus's work on women's power to alter the rape script. It's theoretically potent but has been criticized for the fact that it doesn't deal well with women who "alter" their hearts out and still get raped. See Marcus, "Fighting Bodies, Fighting Words: A Theory and Politics of Rape Prevention," in *Feminists Theorize the Political*, ed. Judith Butler and Joan W. Scott (New York: Routledge, 1992).

[30] Grosz, *Space, Time, and Perversion*, 65.

[31] *FD*, February 8, 1998.

[32] Grosz, *Space, Time, and Perversion*, 89.

[33] All this strife in the face of strong cultural convictions about the badness of fat reminded me, frighteningly, of Judith Butler's reading of the precarious situation of Herculine Barbin, who is the law's embodiment not as "entitled subject, but as an enacted testimony to the law's uncanny capacity to produce only those rebellions that it can guarantee will—out of fidelity—defeat themselves and those subjects who, utterly subjected, have no choice but to reiterate the law of their genesis." *Bodies That Matter*, 106. Though, thankfully, I am not structuralist enough to adopt this stance, it did run through my mind while I was feeling guilty for not being as rebellious as I wanted to be.

[34] Butler, *Excitable Speech*, 2.

[35] Butler, following Foucault, writes that "the paradox of subjectivation . . . is precisely that the subject who would resist such norms is itself enabled, if not produced, by such norms. Although this constitutive constraint does not foreclose the possibility of agency, it does locate agency as a reiterative or rearticulatory practice, immanent to power, and not a relation of external opposition to power." Butler, *Bodies That Matter*, 15.

[36] Butler, *Excitable Speech*, 5.

[37] Butler, *Bodies That Matter*, 193.

[38] Butler's discussion is in regard to "queer." Ibid., 229.

References

Allegra, Donna. "Fat Dancer." In *Journeys to Self-Acceptance: Fat Women Speak*, edited by Carol Wiley, 107–11. Freedom, Calif.: Crossing Press, 1994.

Allon, Natalie. "The Stigma of Overweight in Everyday Life." In *Psychological Aspects of Obesity*, edited by Benjamin B. Wolman, 130–74. New York: Van Nostrand Reinhold, 1982.

Angier, Natalie. "Who Is Fat? It Depends on Culture: Culture and Status." *New York Times*, November 7, 2000, F1.

Anzaldúa, Gloria. *Borderlands/La Frontera: The New Mestiza*. San Francisco: Aunt Lute, 1987.

Bacon, Jane G., and Beatrice E. Robinson. "Fat Phobia and the F-Scale—Measuring, Understanding, and Changing Anti-Fat Attitudes." *Melpomene Journal* 16, no. 1 (Spring 1997): 24+. Available via Responsive Database Services.

Beal, Anne C. "Weighty Matters." *Essence*, January 2001, 123–24.

Beck, Melinda. "An Epidemic of Obesity." *Newsweek*, August 1, 1994, 62–63.

Belkin, Lisa. "Watching Her Weight." *New York Times Magazine*, July 8, 2001, 30–33.

Beller, Anne Scott. *Fat and Thin: A Natural History of Obesity*. New York: Farrar, Straus and Giroux, 1977.

Bernstein, Beth, and Matilda St. John. "The Roseanne Benedict Arnolds." *Bitch: Feminist Response to Pop Culture*, no. 13 (2001): 43–47, 106–7.

Bérubé, Michael. "Foreword: Pressing the Claim." In Simi Linton, *Claiming Disability: Knowledge and Identity*, vii–xi. New York: New York University Press, 1998.

Birmingham, Elizabeth. "Fearing the Freak: How Talk TV Articulates Women and Class." *Journal of Popular Film and Television* 28, no. 3 (Fall 2000): 133+. Available via Responsive Database Services, Inc.

Blank, Hanne. *Big Big Love: A Sourcebook on Sex for People of Size and Those Who Love Them*. Emeryville, Calif.: Greenery Press, 2000.

Bordieu, Pierre. *Distinction: A Social Critique of the Judgment of Taste*. Translated by Richard Nice. Cambridge: Harvard University Press, 1987.

Bordo, Susan. *Unbearable Weight: Feminism, Western Culture, and the Body*. Berkeley: University of California Press, 1993.

Boucher, N. "Overfeds." *New Republic*, September 19, 1994, 36.

Bovey, Shelley. *The Forbidden Body: Why Being Fat Is Not a Sin.* London: Pandora, 1994.

Bray, Rosemary. "Heavy Burden." *Essence*, January 1992, 53–54, 90–91.

Brink, Pamela J. "Fertility and Fat: The Annang Fattening Room." In *Social Aspects of Obesity*, edited by Igor de Garine and Nancy J. Pollock, 71–85. London: Gordon and Breach, 1995.

Brown, Patricia Leigh. "240 Pounds, Persistent and Jazzercise's Equal." *New York Times*, May 8, 2002, A20.

Brown, Roxanne. "Full-Figured Women Fight Back: Resistance Grows to Society's Demand for Slim Bodies." *Ebony*, March 1990, 27–31.

Brown, Suzanne S. "It's Fitting: Fashion Embraces Full-Sized Women." *Denver Post*, November 2, 2000, E1.

Brownfield, Paul. "She's Made Her Case a Bit Too Well." *Los Angeles Times*, June 20, 1999, 8.

Brumberg, Joan Jacobs. *The Body Project: An Intimate History of American Girls.* New York: Random House, 1997.

———. *Fasting Girls: The History of Anorexia Nervosa.* New York: Plume, 1989.

Bryan, T.J. "The Perfect Fit?" *Fireweed* 67, Fat Issue (1999): 38–45.

Burkeman, Oliver. "We're Here and We're Spheres!" *Guardian* (Manchester), August 25, 1998, 7.

Butler, Judith. *Excitable Speech: A Politics of the Performative.* New York: Routledge, 1997.

———. *Bodies That Matter: The Discursive Limits of "Sex."* New York: Routledge, 1993.

———. *Gender Trouble: Feminism and the Subversion of Identity.* New York: Routledge, 1990.

Cahill, Gloria. "Ex-Recluse Turns Shining Star: Actress Darlene Cates Talks about Her New Life in TV and Film." In *Radiance Online: The Magazine for Large Women*, <http://www.radiancemagazine.com/spring95_cahill_cates.html>. Reprinted from Spring 1995 issue; retrieved on October 27, 2000.

Campbell, Jane, and Mike Oliver. *Disability Politics: Understanding Our Past, Changing Our Future.* New York: Routledge, 1996.

Carter, William B. "Health Behavior as a Rational Process: Theory of Reasoned Action and Multiattribute Utility Theory." In *Health Behavior and Health Education: Theory, Research, and Practice*, edited by Karen Glanz, Frances M. Lewis, and Barbara K. Rimer, 63–91. San Francisco: Jossey-Bass, 1990.

Cauvin, Henri E. "South Africa Confronts Another Health Problem: Obesity." *New York Times*, December 19, 2000, F1.

Chapkis, Wendy. "Freaks, Fairies, and Fat Ladies: A Right to Discriminate?" *Critical Sociology* 20, no. 3 (1994): 148–54.

———. *Beauty Secrets: Women and the Politics of Appearance.* Boston: South End Press, 1986.

Clark, Danae. "Commodity Lesbianism." *Camera Obscura* 25, January 1991, 179–201.

Comfort, Alex, ed. *The Joy of Sex: A Gourmet Guide to Love Making.* New York: Fireside Books, 1972.

Cooper, Charlotte. *Fat and Proud: The Politics of Size.* London: Women's Press, 1998.

Crandall, Christian S. "Prejudice against Fat People: Ideology and Self Interest." *Journal of Personality and Social Psychology* 66 (1994): 882–94.

Crandall, Christian S., Silvana D'Anello, Nuray Sakalli, and Eleana Lazarus, Grazyna Wieczorkowska, and N. T. Feather. "An Attribution-Value Model of Prejudice: Anti-Fat Attitudes in Six Nations." *Personality and Social Psychology Bulletin* 27, no. 1 (January 2001): 30–37.

Crisp, A. H. "The Possible Significance of Some Behavioural Correlates of Weight and Carbohydrate Intake." *Journal of Psychosomatic Research* 11, no. 1 (1967): 117.

Cusitar, Leanne, Sherece Taffe, Mariko Tamaki, Allyson Mitchell, Abi Slone, Kerry Daniels-Zraidi, and T. J. Bryan. "Big Fat Editorial." *Fireweed* 67, Fat Issue (Fall 1999): 6–7.

Darke, Paul. "Understanding Cinematic Representations of Disability." In *The Disability Reader: Social Science Perspectives*, edited by Tom Shakespeare, 181–97. London: Cassell, 1998.

Delany, Samuel R. "Street Talk/Straight Talk." *Differences: A Journal of Feminist Cultural Studies* 3, no. 2 (1991): 21–38.

Demarest, Jack, "Body Image: Gender, Ethnic, and Age Differences." *Journal of Social Psychology* 140, no. 4 (August 2000): 465+.

Dolamore, Joan E. "Living Large: The Experiences of Black and White Women of Being Fat in the United States." Ph.D. diss., Harvard University, 1999.

Doty, Alexander. "The Sissy Boy, the Fat Ladies, and the Dykes: Queerness and/as Gender in Pee-wee's World." *Camera Obscura* 25 (January 1991): 125–43.

Douglas, Mary. *Purity and Danger.* New York: Praeger, 1966.

D'Souza, Dinesh. "The National Prospect." *Commentary*, November 1995, 47–48.

Duggan, Lisa. "Making It Perfectly Queer." *Socialist Review* 22, no. 1 (1992): 11–31.

Durgadas, Ganapati S. "Fatness and the Feminized Man." In *Looking Queer: Body Image and Identity in Lesbian, Bisexual, Gay, and Transgender Communities*, edited by Dawn Atkins, 367–71. Binghamton, N.Y.: Haworth, 1998.

Early, Terry. "Ozark Interlude." *Rump Parliament Magazine: Working to Change the Way Society Treats Fat People.* September/October 1994.

Edison, Laurie Toby, and Debbie Notkin. *Women En Large: Images of Fat Nudes.* San Francisco: Books in Focus, 1994.

Edut, Ophira. "Filling Out Fashion—The Expanding Plus-Size Fashion Scene." *Hues,* December 31, 1998, 18.

Edut, Ophira, and Negar Mahmoodzadegan. "The Big Picture: Do Black Women Have Better Body Image Than White Women?" *Hues,* Janurary 31, 1996, 39.

FaT GiRL Publishing. *FaT GiRL: A Zine for Fat Dykes and the Women Who Want Them*, 1. (1994).

Feltz, Vanessa. "Who Says Fat Isn't Sexy?" *Redbook*, December 1993, 45.

Feraios, Andrew J. "If Only I Were Cute: Looksism and Internalized Homophobia in the Gay Male Community." In *Looking Queer: Body Image and Identity in Lesbian, Bisexual, Gay, and Transgender Communities*, edited by Dawn Atkins, 415–29. Binghamton, N.Y.: Haworth, 1998.

Fiedler, Leslie A. "The Tyranny of the Normal." In *The Tyranny of the Normal: An Anthology*, edited by Carol Donley and Sheryl Buckley, 3–10. Kent, Ohio: Kent State University Press, 1996.

Fisher, Seymour. *Body Consciousness: You Are What You Feel*. Englewood Cliffs, N.J.: Prentice-Hall, 1973.

Fitch, Kristine L. "Culture, Ideology, and Interpersonal Communication Research." In *Communication Yearbook* 17, edited by Stan A. Deetz, 104–35. Thousand Oaks, Calif.: Sage, 1994.

Foucault, Michel. *The History of Sexuality, Volume I*. New York: Vintage, 1990.

———. *Discipline and Punish: The Birth of the Prison*. New York: Vintage, 1979.

———. *The Order of Things*. New York: Vintage, 1970.

Fraser, Nancy. "Rethinking the Public Sphere: A Contribution to the Critique of Actually Existing Democracy." In *Habermas and the Public Sphere*, edited by Craig Calhoun, 109–42. Cambridge: MIT Press, 1992.

Fursland, Annie. "Eve Was Framed: Food and Sex and Women's Shame." In *Fed Up and Hungry: Women, Oppression, and Food*, edited by Marilyn Lawrence, 15–26. New York: Peter Bedrick Books, 1987.

Garine, Igor de. "Preface." In *Social Aspects of Obesity*, edited by Garine and Nancy J. Pollock, ix–xi. London: Gordon and Breach, 1995.

———. "Sociocultural Aspects of the Male Fattening Sessions among the Massa of Northern Cameroon." In *Social Aspects of Obesity*, edited by Garine and Nancy J. Pollock, 45–70. London: Gordon and Breach, 1995.

Garland-Thomson, Rosemarie. *Extraordinary Bodies: Figuring Physical Disability in American Culture and Literature*. New York: Columbia University Press, 1997.

Giles, Patrick. "A Matter of Size." In *Looking Queer: Body Image and Identity in Lesbian, Bisexual, Gay, and Transgender Communities*, edited by Dawn Atkins, 355–57. Binghamton, N.Y.: Haworth, 1998.

Gilman, Sander. *Picturing Health and Illness: Images of Identity and Difference*. Baltimore: Johns Hopkins University Press, 1995.

Goldman, Abigail. "Chain Sees Big Business in Larger Sizes: Lane Bryant Has Been Remaking Its Image to Capture More of the Market Catering to 'Realistic Body Sizes.' " *Los Angeles Times*, June 25, 1999, 1.

Goode, Erica. "Watching Volunteers, Experts Seek Clues to Eating Disorders: When Eating Is Disordered." *New York Times*, October 24, 2000, F1.

Goode, Erich, and Joanne Preissler. "Admirers of Fat Women." *Medical Aspects of Human Sexuality* 16, no. 3 (1982): 140–45.

Griffin, Linda Gillan. "Plus Sizes, Plus Style, Plus Profits." *Houston Chronicle*, January 18, 2000, 1.

Grosz, Elizabeth. *Space, Time, and Perversion: Essays on the Politics of Bodies.* New York: Routledge, 1995.

———. *Volatile Bodies: Toward a Corporeal Feminism.* Bloomington: Indiana University Press, 1994.

Gurdon, Meghan Cox. "The Real Skinny on Why We Feel Fat." *Women's Quarterly*, Summer 2000, 29+.

Haravon, Leslie D. "Gaining Respect: Fat Women and Resistance." Ph.D. diss. University of Iowa, 1996.

Haraway, Donna. "The Promise of Monsters: A Regenerative Politics of Inappropriate(d) Others." In *Cultural Studies*, edited by Lawrence Grossberg, Cary Nelson, and Paula A. Treichler, 295–337. New York: Routledge, 1992.

———. "A Manifesto for Cyborgs: Science, Technology, and Socialist Feminism in the 1980s." In *Feminism/Postmodernism*, edited by Linda Nicholson, 190–233. New York: Routledge, 1990.

Harris, M. B., L. C. Walters, and S. Waschull. "Gender and Ethnic Differences in Obesity-Related Behaviors and Attitudes in a College Sample." *Journal of Applied Social Psychology* 21 (1991): 1545–77.

Hicks, Chris. "Movie Review: What's Eating Gilbert Grape." On Deseret News website, <http://deseretnews.com/movies/view/1,1257,1994,00.html>. Reviewed on March 4, 1994; retrieved on October 27, 2000.

Hinden, Pam. "The Fats of Life: Reflections on the Tyranny of Fatophobia." *Off Our Backs: A Women's Newsjournal*, March 31, 1983: 30.

Huspek, Michael. "Dueling Structures: The Theory of Resistance in Discourse." *Communication Theory* 3, no. 1 (1993): 1–25.

Jeffery, R. W. "Minnesota Studies on Community-Based Approaches to Weight Loss and Control." *Annals of Internal Medicine* 119, no. 7 (October 1 1993), pt. 2: 719–21.

Johansson, Warren, and William A. Percy. *Outing: Shattering the Conspiracy of Silence.* New York: Haworth, 1994.

Kaiser, Amy. "Safety in Pounds." *Moxie*, Summer 1999. Available from Contemporary Women's Issues Database via Responsive Database Services.

Kampf, Ray. *The Bear Handbook: A Comprehensive Guide for Those Who Are Husky, Hairy, and Homosexual and Those Who Love 'Em.* New York: Harrington Park, 2000.

Kane, Courtney. "A Male Sex Symbol Enjoys the Company of Larger Women in a New Campaign for Lane Bryant." *New York Times*, February 1, 2001, C8.

Keating, Erin. "What's the Big Deal? Erin Keating Reflects on the Bold 'n' Fleshy Frontier of *Mode* Magazine." *Bitch: Feminist Response to Pop Culture* 3, no. 2 (July 1998): 34.

Kennedy, Angela. "Fair Deal? Fat Chance." *Nursing Standard* 9, no. 21 (February 15, 1995): 45.

Klein, Richard. *Eat Fat.* New York: Pantheon, 1996.

———. "Big Country." *New Republic*, September 19, 1994, 28–37.

Klug, Foster. "Triathlete Won't Let Fat Get in the Way of Fit." *Los Angeles Times*, January 28, 2001, B4.

Kolata, Gina. "While Children Grow Fatter, Experts Search for Solutions: Learning to Eat." *New York Times*, October 19, 2000, A1.

———. "The Burdens of Being Overweight: Mistreatment and Misconceptions." *New York Times*, November 22, 1992, A1.

Kotler, Philip. *Marketing for Nonprofit Organizations.* Englewood Cliffs, N.J.: Prentice-Hall, 1982.

Kozloff, Arielle P., and David Gordon Mitten. *The Gods Delight: The Human Figure in Classical Bronze.* Cleveland: Cleveland Museum of Art, 1988.

Kuczynksi, Alex. "The Incredible Shrinking Plus-Size Model." *New York Times*, March 29, 1998, sec. 9, 4.

LaFollette, Laetitia. Telephone interview by author. Amherst, Massachusetts. November 20, 1994.

Lamm, Nomy. "Fashion: I Love Dressing Up." *Ms.*, April/May 1999, 12.

———. "Fishnets, Feather Boas, and Fat." In *Adiós, Barbie: Young Women Write about Body Image and Identity*, edited by Ophira Edut, 78–87. Seattle: Seal Press, 1998.

"Large and in Charge: Full-Figured Celebrities Proud of Their Stature." *Jet*, April 17, 2000, 52–57.

Levine, Michelle Joy. *I Wish I Were Thin, I Wish I Were Fat.* New York: Fireside Books, 1999.

Linton, Simi. *Claiming Disability: Knowledge and Identity.* New York: New York University Press, 1998.

Louderback, Llewellyn. *Fat Power: Whatever You Weigh Is Right.* New York: Hawthorn, 1970.

Manheim, Camryn. "If We're All a Little Pudgier in 2025, So What?" *Time*, November 8, 1999, 90.

———. *Wake Up! I'm Fat!* New York: Broadway Books, 1999.

Mann, G. V. "The Influence of Obesity on Health." *New England Journal of Medicine* 291 (1974): 178–85.

Mann, Patricia S. *Micropolitics: Agency in a Postfeminist Era.* Minneapolis: University of Minnesota, 1994.

Manton, Catherine. *Fed Up: Women and Food in America.* Westport, Conn.: Bergin and Garvey, 1999.

Marcus, Sharon. "Fighting Bodies, Fighting Words: A Theory and Politics of Rape Prevention." In *Feminists Theorize the Political*, edited by Judith Butler and Joan W. Scott, 385–403. New York: Routledge, 1992.

Maringer, Johannes, and Hans-Georg Bandi. *Art in the Ice Age.* New York: Praeger, 1953.

McCrea, Celia, and Maurice Yaffe. "Sexuality in the Obese." *British Journal of Sexual Medicine* 8, no. 69 (February 1981): 24, 34–37.

McFarland, Barbara, and Tyeis Baker-Baumann. "Shame and Body Image: Culture and the Compulsive Eater." In *The Tyranny of the Normal: An An-*

thology, edited by Carol Donley and Sheryl Buckley, 89–110. Kent, Ohio: Kent State University Press, 1996.

McKinley, Nita M. "Ideal Weight/Ideal Women: Society Constructs the Female." In *Weighty Issues: Fatness and Thinness as Social Problems*, edited by Jeffery Sobal and Donna Maurer, 97–115. New York: Aldine de Gruyter, 1999.

Medina, José F., Joel Saegert, and Alicia Gresham. "Comparison of Mexican-American and Anglo-American Attitudes toward Money." *Journal of Consumer Affairs* 30 (Summer 1996): 124–45.

Merrett, Jim. "The Size of the Matter: After Years of Being Settled For, Big Men Come into Their Own." *Advocate*, October 22, 1991, 60–61.

Miller, Carol T., Esther D. Rothblum, Diane Felicio, and Pamela Brand. "Compensating for Stigma: Obese and Nonobese Women's Reactions to Being Visible." *Personality and Social Psychology Bulletin* 21, no. 10 (October 1995): 1093–106.

National Association to Advance Fat Acceptance. *NAAFA Newsletter*, October/November 1994 and December 1994/January 1995.

Nichter, Mimi. *Fat Talk: What Girls and Their Parents Say about Dieting*. Cambridge: Harvard University Press, 2000.

NIH Technology Assessment Conference Panel. "Methods for Voluntary Weight Loss and Control." *Annals of Internal Medicine* 119, no. 7 (October 1, 1993), part 2: 764–70.

Notkin, Debbie. "Enlarging: Politics and Society." In Laurie Toby Edison and Notkin, *Women En Large: Images of Fat Nudes*, 91–107. San Francisco: Books in Focus, 1994.

———. Interview by author. Northampton, Mass., November 16, 1994.

Ogden, Jane. *Fat Chance! The Myth of Dieting Explained*. London: Routledge, 1992.

Orbach, Susie. *Hunger Strike*. London: Faber and Faber, 1986.

———. *Fat Is a Feminist Issue*. New York: Berkley Books, 1978.

Patton, Cindy. "Tremble, Hetero Swine!" In *Fear of a Queer Planet: Queer Politics and Social Theory*, edited by Michael Warner, 143–77. Minneapolis: University of Minnesota Press, 1993.

Peterman, Erika D. "A Big Idea Catches On: Trendy Clothes in Plus Sizes." *Los Angeles Times*, November 19, 1999, 1.

Peters, Susan. "The Politics of Disability Identity." In *Disability and Society: Emerging Issues and Insights*, edited by Len Barton, 215–34. New York: Addison Wesley Longman, 1996.

Pinkwater, Daniel. "I'm Going to Say It!" *Rump Parliament Magazine: Working to Change the Way Society Treats Fat People*, September 1994.

Pi-Sunyer, F. Xavier. "Medical Hazards of Obesity." *Annals of Internal Medicine* 119, no. 7 (October 1, 1993), pt. 2: 655–60.

Pollock, Nancy J. "Social Fattening Patterns in the Pacific—The Positive Side of Obesity. A Nauru Case Study." In *Social Aspects of Obesity*, edited by Igor de Garine and Pollock, 87–109. London: Gordon and Breach, 1995.

Pool, Robert. *FAT: Fighting the Obesity Epidemic*. New York: Oxford, 2001.

Powter, Susan. *Stop the Insanity!* New York: Simon and Schuster, 1993.

"Public Health: America's Getting Fatter." *American Journal of Nursing* 94, no. 9 (1994): 9.

Quinn, Diane M., and Jennifer Crocker. "When Ideology Hurts: Effects of Belief in the Protestant Ethic and Feeling Overweight on the Psychological Well-Being of Women." *Journal of Personality and Social Psychology* 77, no. 2 (August 1999): 402–14.

Rand, Colleen S. W. "Obesity and Human Sexuality." *Medical Aspects of Human Sexuality* 13, no. 1 (1979): 141–52.

Ridgway, Mindy. "Fat Dykes on Fat Dykes: Hot off the Press." *San Francisco Bay Times*, October 6, 1994, 6–7, 17.

Rosenstock, Irwin M. "The Health Belief Model: Explaining Health Behavior through Expectancies." In *Health Behavior and Health Education: Theory, Research, and Practice*, edited by Karen Glanz, Frances M. Lewis, and Barbara K. Rimer, 39–62. San Francisco: Jossey-Bass, 1990.

Rosin, Hanna. "Solid Citizens." *New Republic*, September 19, 1994, 26.

Rubin, Gayle S. "Thinking Sex: Notes for a Radical Theory of the Politics of Sexuality." In *Pleasure and Danger: Exploring Female Sexuality*, edited by Carole S. Vance, 267–319. Boston: Routledge and Kegan Paul, 1984.

Rubin, Sylvia. " 'The View's' Star Jones Shares Her Fashion Savvy." *San Francisco Chronicle*, May 9, 2000, E6.

Rucker, C. E., III, and T. F. Cash. "Body Images, Body Size Perceptions, and Eating Behavior among African-American and White College Women." *International Journal of Eating Disorders* 12 (1992): 291–99.

Russo, Mary. *The Female Grotesque: Risk, Excess, and Modernity*. London: Routledge, 1995.

Safire, William. "All Phat! and a Bag of Chips." *New York Times Magazine*, May 17, 1998, 30.

Schoenfielder, Lisa, and Barb Wieser, eds. *Shadow on a Tightrope: Writings by Women on Fat Oppression*. San Francisco: Aunt Lute, 1983.

Schulman, Sarah. *My American History: Lesbian and Gay Life during the Reagan/Bush Years*. New York: Routledge, 1994.

Schur, Edwin M. *The Politics of Deviance: Stigma Contests and the Uses of Power*. Englewood Cliffs, N.J.: Prentice-Hall, 1980.

Schwartz, Hillel. *Never Satisfied: A Cultural History of Diets, Fantasies, and Fat*. New York: Free Press, 1986.

Scott, Sophfronia, and Ulrica Wihlborg. "Finishing Touches." *People Weekly*, June 17, 2002, 96–102.

Sedgwick, Eve Kosofsky. "Epistemology of the Closet." In *The Lesbian and Gay Studies Reader*, edited by Henry Abelove, Michèle Aina Barale, and David M. Halperin, 45–61. New York: Routledge, 1993.

Sedgwick, Eve Kosofsky, and Michael Moon. "Divinity: A Dossier, a Performance Piece, a Little-Understood Emotion." In Eve Kosofsky Sedgwick, *Tendencies*, 215–51. Durham, N.C.: Duke University Press, 1993.

Shilling, Chris. *The Body and Social Theory*. London: Sage, 1993.

"ShopKo's Plus-Plus (Size) Situation." *DSN Retailing Today* 39, no. 18 (2000): A8–A10.

Siegfried, Michael L. "The Inner City in the 21st Century: Huxley's Brave New World Revisited." *Journal of Interdisciplinary Studies* 8, nos. 1–2 (1996): 19–30.

Skenazy, Lenore. "Extra Fares for Fat Folk are Flighty." *New York Daily News*, June 26, 2002, 33.

Smith, Craig S. "Risking Limbs for Height, and Success, in China," *New York Times*, May 5, 2002, A3.

Sobo, Elisa J. "The Sweetness of Fat: Health, Procreation, and Sociability in Rural Jamaica." In *Many Mirrors: Body Image and Social Relations*, edited by Nicole Sault, 132–54. New Brunswick, N.J.: Rutgers University Press, 1994.

Solovay, Sondra. *Tipping the Scales of Justice: Fighting Weight-Based Discrimination*. Amherst, N.Y.: Prometheus, 2000.

Spelman, Elizabeth V. *Inessential Woman: Problems of Exclusion in Feminist Thought*. Boston: Beacon, 1990.

Spitzack, Carole. *Confessing Excess: Women and the Politics of Body Reduction*. Albany: State University of New York Press, 1990.

Stewart, Andrew. *Greek Sculpture: An Exploration*. 2 vols. New Haven: Yale University Press, 1990.

Stewart, John. *Bridges Not Walls: A Book about Interpersonal Communication*. 7th ed. New York: McGraw-Hill, 1999.

Steyn, Mark. "Obestiality: America Has the Weight of Its Weight on Its Shoulders." *American Spectator* 31, 54–56. Available at <http://www.spectator.org/archives/98-03_steyn.html>.

Stinson, Susan. *Belly Songs: In Celebration of Fat Women*. Northampton, Mass.: Orogeny Press, 1993.

Sullivan, Andrew. "The Plump Classes Are on a Roll." *Sunday Times* (London), August 29, 1999. Full text available via LexisNexis.

Teti, Victor. "Food and Fatness in Calabria." Translated by Nicollete S. James. In *Social Aspects of Obesity*, edited by Igor de Garine and Nancy J. Pollock, 3–29. London: Gordon and Breach, 1995.

Textor, Alex Robertson. "Organization, Specialization, and Desires in the Big Men's Movement: Preliminary Research in the Study of Subculture-Formation." *Journal of Gay, Lesbian, and Bisexual Identity* 4, no. 3 (July 1999): 217–39.

Thompson, Becky Wangsgaard. " 'A Way Outa No Way': Eating Problems among African-American, Latina, and White Women." *Gender and Society* 6, no. 4 (1992): 546–61.

Thone, Ruth Raymond. *Fat—A Fate Worse Than Death? Women, Weight and Appearance*. New York: Haworth, 1997.

Travis, Michelle A. "Perceived Disabilities, Social Cognition, and 'Innocent Mistakes.' " *Vanderbilt Law Review*, March 2002, 55 Vand. L. Rev 481. Available via LexisNexis.

Turner, Victor. *The Ritual Process*. Ithaca: Cornell University Press, 1977.

Urgo, Marisa, for the Office of Minority Health–U.S. Department of Health and Human Services. "Closing the Gap" (1998): 6. Available via Responsive Database Services.

Valente, Marcela. "Rights–Argentina: Legislating Larger Clothing Sizes for Women." *Interpress Service* (newsletter), March 8, 2000. Full text available from Contemporary Women's Issues database via Responsive Database Services, Inc.

Walker, Roxy. "The Next Generation of Activists: Frank, Thoughtful, Articulate." *Radiance: The Magazine for Large Women*, Summer 1995, 8.

Wallack, Lawrence. "Media Advocacy: Promoting Health through Mass Communication." In *Health Behavior and Health Education: Theory, Research, and Practice*, edited by Karen Glanz, Frances M. Lewis, and Barbara K. Rimer, 370–86. San Francisco: Jossey-Bass, 1990.

Walton, Amy. "Fat Girl Walking." *Fireweed* 67, Fat Issue (1999): 56–57.

Wann, Marilyn. "Women: Self-Hatred and Celery Sticks. Life Is Too Short for Either." *Guardian* (Manchester), March 29, 1999, T007. Available via ProQuest.

———. *Fat! So? Because You Don't Have to Apologize for Your Size!* Berkeley, Calif.: Ten Speed Press, 1998.

Weeks, Janet. "Activists Plan a 'No-Diet Day.' " *St. Louis Post Dispatch*, May 2, 1994, 4D.

White, Randall. *Dark Caves, Bright Visions: Life in Ice Age Europe*. New York: Norton, 1986.

Williams, Regina D. "Conquering the Fear of a Fat Body: The Journey toward Myself." In *Adiós, Barbie: Young Women Write about Body Image and Identity*, edited by Ophira Edut, 176–87. Seattle: Seal Press, 1998.

Willmuth, Mary. "Treatment of Obesity: A Socio-Political Perspective." *Women and Therapy* 5, no. 4 (December 31, 1986): 27.

Winter, Greg. "Fraudulent Marketers Capitalize on Demand for Sweat-Free Diets." *New York Times*, October 29, 2000, sec. 1, 1.

Wise, Jonathan, and Susan Kierr Wise. *The Overeaters: Eating Styles and Personality*. New York: Human Sciences Press, 1979.

Wittig, Monique. *The Straight Mind and Other Essays*. Boston: Beacon Press, 1992.

Wolf, Naomi. *The Beauty Myth*. New York: Doubleday, 1991.

Wright, Les. *The Bear Book: Readings in the History and Evolution of a Gay Male Subculture*. New York: Haworth, 1997.

"Your Momma Jokes." Available at <http://www.yourmom.com>; accessed January 18, 2001.

Index

abjection, 3, 5, 28, 68, 98, 124, 139n. 2
activism: related to clothing, 68–69, 72; queer, 89
actresses, 41, 43. *See also* Burke, Delta; Garofalo, Janeane; Jones, Star; Lake, Ricki; Manheim, Camryn; Najimy, Kathy; Queen Latifah; Roseanne; Winfrey, Oprah
ACT-Up, 89, 95
advertising, 66–67, 71, 101, 107; gay window, 71
affinity politics, 2, 8–9, 11, 107, 110; queer, 13
Africa, North, concepts of fatness in, 21–23
African Americans, 27, 35, 42–43, 46, 59–62, 113, 134n. 43. *See also* blacks; race
Afro-Caribbean culture, 62
age, 66
agency, 2–3, 5, 14, 99, 108, 110, 116–17
Alafonte, Chupoo, 47
alienation, 52
Allegra, Donna, 59
American Cancer Society, 30
American Dream, 56
American Public Health Association, 37
American Spectator, 111
Americans with Disabilities Act, 75, 116
Anderson, Louie, 75
Andrew, Alexa, 62
Angier, Natalie, 113
animalism, 86

Annang, 22
anonymity, 103
anorexia, 15, 66, 127n. 21. *See also* eating disorders
anxiety, 31
Aphrodite, 19–20, 128n. 32
appetite, 87–88
Argentina, 67
armrests, 117
Arnold, Roseanne. *See* Roseanne
art, 127n. 24
arthritis, 30
Asian Americans, 46
assimilationism, 42–47, 52, 72, 89, 111–12, 130–31n. 4
athletes, tri-, 112

Bandi, Hans-Georg, 17
Banzas, Maria del Carmen, 66, 135n. 11
Barbin, Herculine, 142n. 33
Barr, Roseanne. *See* Roseanne
Bear Book, The, 91
Bear Handbook, 91
bears, 90–91
beauty: and citizenship, 55; differing historical and cultural concepts of, 1, 5, 15, 19–20, 21, 23, 58, 65, 98, 131n. 31; ideologies of, 3, 6–8, 25, 50–53, 59, 68, 76, 80; industry, 71; pageants, 68; as political, 63; and sexuality, 40–41, 46–47; of thinness, 86
Beauvoir, Simone de, 11
behavior modification, 31

Born in Miami and raised primarily in upstate New York, KATHLEEN LEBESCO received her B.A. and M.A. in Communication and Rhetoric from the University of Albany, State University of New York, and her Ph.D. in Communication from the University of Massachusetts Amherst. She is associate professor of communication arts at Marymount Manhattan College and resides in Westchester County, N.Y. LeBesco teaches classes in communication history and theory, popular culture, feminist and queer theory, and food studies and has received multiple teaching awards. She is coeditor of *Bodies Out of Bounds: Fatness and Transgression* and *The Drag King Anthology* and received a top competitive paper award from the Disability Caucus of the National Communication Association.